2

Praise for the First

Ronnie Lott, Fox Sports, former NFL star

"I was happy to contribute to this book because it's packed with vital information about what it takes to succeed in sports, school, and, more importantly, life."

Rick Telander, *ESPN The Magazine*

"Complete, comprehensive, and easy to read. A great benefit to any young athlete considering playing sports in college."

Dale Brown, former college basketball coach

"If you're interested in becoming eligible, read the NCAA Guide. If you're interested in getting a meaningful education, read this book."

Bill Walton, NBC Sports, former NBA star

"This book reveals the inner workings of college sports so that athletes can take charge of their lives. Our young people are in trouble. Parents should read this desperately needed book to help their kids."

Janet M. Justus, former NCAA Director of Education Outreach

"Excellent insights into recruitment, including rarely stated truths: a must-read for prospective student-athletes."

Dr. Kathleen Gabriel, academic advisor, University of Arizona

"Athletes must prepare for college success in high school. This book shows them how—in an entertaining, inspiring way."

Darrin Nelson, assistant athletic director, Stanford University

"Every potential student-athlete should read this book prior to picking a college or university. This is one of life's most important decisions; the book helps athletes choose a place and setting where they will be happy and productive and not just consider sports. I will definitely have my sons read this guide when they reach college age."

Bob Corb, Ph.D., sports psychologist

"Finally, a book for student-athletes and their parents that cuts through the hype to address the real issues. Read this book before you make any decisions about college."

Joel Corry, sports agent

"If an athlete doesn't want to be exploited or taken advantage of, the first step is to read this book. Then they need to take action."

Bob Bender,
head basketball coach, University of Washington

"This book is right on target. It helps athletes make informed decisions about all the critical issues they face from the time they enter high school through their college years and beyond."

Joseph Halper,
former Commissioner of Recreation of New York City

"The writing and the cartoons express key points in a way that high school and college athletes will enjoy."

Krista Blomquist, pro beach volleyball player

"This book is an excellent motivational tool for high school and college athletes who want to succeed. The book tells you exactly what you need to know and what actions you need to take."

Bill Donlon, basketball coach, Lake Forest High School

"I've been involved in high school and college basketball as an athlete, coach, and parent. This book sets forth outstanding guidelines for recruiting and preparation for college."

Jerry Wainwright,
head basketball coach, University of North Carolina–Wilmington

"This is the most comprehensive guide to recruiting ever written. Must reading for prospective student-athletes and their families—and even coaches."

Dan Kreft, pro basketball player and Web site designer

"If this book had been around when I was in high school, it would have saved me a lot of grief."

Chris Myers, Fox Sports

"After years of interviewing athletes, I have found that the ones who are the most grounded understand self-accountability. This book teaches this important lesson."

Eric Allen, NFL Pro Bowl cornerback

"This book provides a tremendous game plan for high school and college athletes to succeed on the field and in the classroom. You know if Ronnie Lott is involved, it's going to be first-rate."

THE STUDENT ATHLETE SURVIVAL GUIDE

Marc Isenberg and Rick Rhoads

Ragged Mountain Press / McGraw-Hill

Camden, Maine • New York • San Francisco • Washington, D.C.
Auckland • Bogotá • Caracas • Lisbon • London • Madrid
Mexico City • Milan • Montreal • New Delhi • San Juan • Singapore
Sydney • Tokyo • Toronto

Ragged Mountain Press

A Division of The McGraw·Hill Companies

2 4 6 8 10 9 7 5 3 1

Library of Congress Cataloging-in-Publication Data
Isenberg, Marc, 1967–
The student-athlete survival guide / Marc Isenberg and Rick Rhoads.
p.   cm.
Includes bibliographical references (p.   ) and index.
ISBN 0-07-136442-0
1. High school athletes—Education—United States. 2. College athletes—Education—United States. 3. High school athletes—United States—Life skills guides. 4. College athletes—United States—Life skills guide. I. Rhoads, Rick. II. Title.

LC2581.I84 2000
378.1'98—dc21   00-055268

Questions regarding the content of this book should be addressed to
Ragged Mountain Press
P.O. Box 220
Camden, ME 04843
www.raggedmountainpress.com

Questions regarding the ordering of this book should be addressed to
The McGraw-Hill Companies
Customer Service Department
P.O. Box 547
Blacklick, OH 43004
Retail customers: 1-800-262-4729
Bookstores: 1-800-722-4726

Printed on 60 lb. Computer Book by R. R. Donnelley, Crawfordsville, IN
Design by Joyce C. Weston
Production by PerfecType, Nashville, TN
Production Coordination by Dan Kirchoff
Edited by Tom McCarthy and Cynthia Flanagan Goss

AUTHORS' NOTE: This guide is designed to provide accurate and authoritative information in regard to the subject matter covered. It is sold with the understanding that the authors are not engaged in rendering legal, financial, or other professional advice or services. If legal, financial, or other expert assistance is required, the services of a competent professional should be sought.

To my grandfather, Alfred (Babe) Holtz,
for giving me the confidence to make this book a reality.

—MARC ISENBERG

In memory of my Dad, Professor Lester Rhoads,
a real athlete and a real scholar.

—RICK RHOADS

Contents

Part 4. The College Years

List of Cartoons

Acknowledgments

In May 1994, I went to UCLA to research a freelance article. Wayne Johnson, who worked in the UCLA Athletic Department, arranged for me to speak with over fifty athletes. I was blown away by the knowledge and insight of this group, which included Ed O'Bannon, Tyus Edney, George Zidek, Toby Bailey, "JR" Henderson, Lisa Fernandez, Karim Abdul-Jabbar, J. J. Stokes, and Donnie Edwards. They gave me the idea and the motivation to write this book. They inspired me to ask questions and talk to many more people—athletes, coaches, parents, counselors, administrators, and psychologists. This in turn led to a memorable four-hour interview with legendary UCLA coach John Wooden.

The number of people who contributed to this book began to add up. If you find *The Student-Athlete Survival Guide* useful, it's because so many people generously shared their time and wisdom. Rick Rhoads and I would like to say thank you to those who contributed.

I'd like first to thank my mom and dad, whose love and support never wavered.

Thanks to the A-Game.com Advisory Board of Dale Brown, Allen Sack, Arnie Wexler, Janet Justus, Doug Single, Jeff Fellenzer, Maidie Oliveau, Joel Corry, and Bob Corb, for their guidance and action. Ronnie Lott, Ann Meyers Drysdale, and Mike "Coach K" Krzyzewski, thank you for believing in this project and lending your time and names to this book. Sebastian Conley, it was a pleasure to work with you as you transformed our ideas into cartoons; you got the message—and added to it. Dan Kreft, thank you for your design of the original Web site, and for your slam-dunk editing. Without the proofreading of Katy Leclercq and Peggy Rhoads, our message about attention to detail might have lost credibility.

The people at the Amateur Athletic Foundation, including Anita DeFrantz, Mike Salmon, and Wayne Wilson, provided a meeting place and research support. People who work in the trenches as academic advisors—such as Kathleen Gabriel, Jack Rivas, and Wayne Johnson—never get the credit they deserve for the work they do with student-athletes; their contribution to this book was invaluable. Steve Mallonee of the NCAA and Kevin Henry of the NAIA helped ensure the technical accuracy of this guide. UCLA compliance officer Rich Herczog guided us through the complexities of the NCAA and financial aid. Bob Corb contributed his expertise to the section on sports psychology. Thanks to our publishers, Tom McCarthy and Jon Eaton at Ragged Mountain Press. Great people (who happen to also be great athletes) we've met along the way—including Jameel Pugh, Shane Battier, Mark Madsen, "TJ" Cummings, Marcus Taylor, Josh Pastner, Stephanie Wasserman, Krista Blomquist, Lisa Griffith, Tennille Grant, Chris Johnson, Anya Kolbisen, Antawn Jamison, and Riza Manning—shared their experiences on A-Game.com and helped bring this book to life.

Other people whose involvement was invaluable include: Tim McCormick, Purvis Short, Stacey Robinson, Ian Bjorhovde, Rich Goodnight, Robert Sax, Vince Carter, Fred Claire, Frank Dubois, Art Dye, Murray Sperber, Andrew Zimbalist, Randy Harvey, Steve Hartman, Dewey Knudson, Jeff Moeller, Tubby Smith, Joe Paterno, Debbie Spander, Wendy Spander, Leigh Steinberg, Gene Washington, Mike Bantam, Bill Walton, Rick Telander, Mitch Kupchak, Holly McPeak, Bob Costas, Brian Taylor, Chris Myers, Keenan McCardell, Eric Allen, Bob Bender, Jeff Fellenzer, Shantay Legans, Larry and Renee Anenberg, Tom Hoffarth, Ann Victor, Mike Murray, Bob Ibach, Barry Temkin, Darrin Nelson, Mike Wimmer, Steve Appel, Victoria Wood, Linda Tobin, Katrina Lemke, Sue Levine, Kristin Hughes, Bill Bennett, Marty Anenberg, Jackie Hamlett, Rob Miech, Marques Johnson, Nick Zaccagnino, Milt and Avis Henderson, John Bailey, Donald Dell, Ralph Jackson, Mike Izzi, Quin Snyder, Sonny Vaccaro, Brentt Eads, Andy Bark, George Raveling, Steve Krone, Jerry Wainwright, Bill and Mary Ann Donlon, Shirley Ito, Risa Gordon, Deirdre Leclercq, Bob and Doris Leclercq, Al Hergott, Peter Rudman, Marv Auerbach—and many more.

Marc Isenberg
marc@a-game.com

THE /A game Way

Put school first, sports second.

Understand that sports are not forever and that education will secure my future.

Play to win, but not at all costs.

Work on fundamentals without coaches' orders.

Study even when no assignment is due.

Don't cheat, or participate in cheating, even if I know I can get away with it.

Read and think.

Trust people who earn my trust.

Understand that learning from failure is part of the journey to success.

Set goals and make plans to reach them.

Accept responsibility, don't make excuses, and deliver what I promise.

Don't do drugs or steroids.

Know right from wrong.

Keep my sense of humor!

Reality Checks

This Book Won't Work Unless You Do

Success does not come from quick fixes or magic potions. This book tells you what has worked for other athletes . . . and what hasn't. It's up to you to apply these principles.

South Coast Doesn't Exist

To illustrate key points, we describe events in the lives of several athletes and coaches. The problems are real, but the characters are fictitious. We also write about the inner workings of the Athletic Department at South Coast State University. This school doesn't exist, nor does its arch rival, North Coast. A parent who read a draft of this book asked us for the phone number of the South Coast volleyball coach. After a miserable recruiting experience, the athlete's father thought "Kelly Hughes," whose story begins on page 57, would be the ideal coach for his daughter. Although we had to explain that we had invented the whole thing, we're pleased it sounded so real.

This Book Doesn't Rule Sports

We're confident that *The Student-Athlete Survival Guide* is the authoritative book on its subject. We've interviewed hundreds of athletes, parents, coaches, academic advisors, compliance officers, and NCAA, NAIA, and NJCAA officials to be sure we're giving you correct information. But, as much as we might like it to, this book doesn't govern college sports. The groups with the initials do. The NCAA rule book is ten times as thick as this book (and 1,000 times less readable). The rules change every year. So if you need to clarify a particular point, please check with the NCAA, the Initial-Eligibility Clearinghouse, or with the many knowledgeable experts dedicated to serving student athletes. If you're dealing with a college governed by the NAIA or NJCAA, check with them. If you screw up, no governing body will accept as a defense, "*The Student-Athlete Survival Guide* said I could do it."

Pregame

by Ronnie Lott

Let me tell you a story to show why *The Student-Athlete Survival Guide* can make a big difference in your life.

During my freshman year at the University of Southern California (USC), I was put into a game for one play with instructions to do nothing but cover the tight end. Instead, I tried to sack the quarterback. I wanted to be the hero. I was within inches of the quarterback when he completed a 1-yard touchdown pass to the wide-open tight end. The extra point put our arch rival, the University of California–Los Angeles (UCLA) up 27–26 with two minutes to play. Fortunately we kicked a last-second field goal to win the game.

I had ignored my assignment and acted as if I knew more than the coach. It was a devastating mistake, but I was determined not to let one play ruin my career. Every day that summer I went to my high school practice field. I lined up in front of an imaginary tight end and covered him in every defense USC used. It had to look crazy to anyone who was watching, but I was determined to prove that I could be counted on. What can you learn from this story?

- **You are responsible for your success.** If you want something, do all the things, large and small, necessary to attain it. I'm talking about success as an athlete, and, even more importantly, as a student and all-around person.
- **Everyone makes mistakes.** Don't be afraid to make mistakes—and don't make excuses. Face up to your mistakes and learn from them, or you cannot succeed.
- **Don't get burned by your ego.** I had been taught to sacrifice my individual wishes for the good of the team. But against UCLA I tried to be a star instead of focusing on what the team needed from me.

Never underestimate how far these ideas can take you. They certainly helped my teammates on the San Francisco 49ers. Many so-called experts said that Joe Montana wasn't big enough to be a quarterback and didn't have a strong enough arm. They said Jerry Rice couldn't make the transition from Mississippi Valley State football to the pros.

They said I was too small to be an NFL safety. But the 49ers went on to win four Super Bowls in the 1980s.

What Does It Take to Succeed?

Everybody in the 49er organization knew his role and took personal responsibility for helping the team win. Ownership and management were the best in the League. They made sure we had all the tools necessary to win, from a state-of-the-art training facility to charter flights to away games. They provided the resources for the coaches and general manager to get the best talent. Head Coach Bill Walsh took a total business approach to winning, from long-range strategy to the smallest detail. Our players looked for every advantage to gain the upper hand: conditioning, off-season training, nutrition, mind exercises. If you convinced some 49ers that their play would improve if they wore lipstick, the next day at practice you'd see a lot of guys sporting shiny red lips. To be a 49er you had to be committed to doing all the large and small things necessary to achieve excellence.

When people made mistakes, our attitude was neither to blame nor excuse. We used the mistake to learn how to do it right next time.

If your attitude was, "Look at me, I'm a great football player!" you didn't fit into the 49ers. On the field, we blocked out distractions such as money issues and the media. We respected ourselves and each other because we focused on the basics that got us to the top: hard work and perseverance.

Another team might have been bigger, stronger, or faster—on paper. We didn't care. Life is not about how you measure up on paper, whether it's your 40-yard time or your SAT score. It's about wanting something bad enough to do what it takes to get it. My teammates knew I would go to war for them in every game.

Dumb-Jock Myth

To be a success, you have to get an education. Most athletes are not going to make their living from their sport after college. That's just the reality. Statistically, you have a better chance of becoming a brain surgeon than a professional athlete.

When I arrived at USC, I promised myself that I would get my degree. I did not buy into the dumb-jock myth. You have to be disciplined, competitive, and smart to excel as an athlete. These are the same qualities you need to succeed in the classroom.

Why go to college and not graduate? Too often athletes look at college as simply a step to the pros. It's OK to dream that you will make the big time. But if you are smart and realistic, you understand that your dream might not pan out. I remember being so tired after practice that I had to force myself to go to the library, force myself to open a book, and force myself to concentrate. I knew that if I tried to just get by in the classroom, sooner or later it would catch up with me.

To be a success, you have to get help from others. I was fortunate to have parents, coaches, and teachers who supported my goals and dreams and gave me guidance and instilled discipline. I purposely surrounded myself with friends who were motivated to succeed and who supported each other.

Who Do I Want to Become?

Every day, on TV or in the newspapers, you hear about college or professional athletes who have committed crimes, become addicted to drugs or alcohol, abused women, or become involved with illegal gambling. Why do these athletes risk their careers, freedom, and health? It's not because they are happy and secure. Something is out of balance in their lives. Despite their success in sports, these athletes are not satisfied—and they become their own worst enemies.

When you know who you are and where you want to go, it's easier to decide what to do. But when we're so busy practicing our sport or meeting other time-consuming demands, we forget to take stock of our values. When that happens, we risk making decisions that hurt our chances to get what we really want out of life. All of us need to step back once in a while and ask ourselves, "Who am I, and who do I want to become?" As a young person, these questions are especially important for you: most of your life is still ahead of you.

Use this book to help you get the edge that will make you a success in sports, school, and everything you do.

NFL Hall of Fame member **Ronnie Lott** won four Super Bowls with the San Francisco 49ers. A commentator for Fox Sports, he is the cofounder of Champion Ventures, a firm that invests in high-tech companies.

PART ONE

The Road To Success

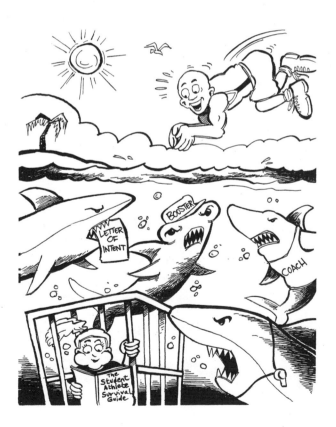

CHAPTER 1

Bring Your A-Game

Tiger Woods said, "When I bring my A-game, I'm tough to beat." Toronto Raptor star Vince Carter said, "I'm going to have to step up and play because Grant Hill is going to bring his A-game." *A-game* is used so frequently in sports to refer to top performance that it has become a cliché. Few people stop to think that the *A* in A-game comes from the classroom.

Excellent students earn their *A* grades by consistent study. Similarly, excellent athletes put themselves in position to "bring their A-game" by consistent preparation, including practice, training, attention to nutrition and health—all the ingredients that go in to maximizing performance. The goal of this book is to help you play your A-game, in school and in sports.

The A-Game Approach to Success

For athletes, participating in sports is a vital part of life. In sports, you can develop intelligence and fitness, integrity, and friendships. You can learn skills—physical, social, and intellectual—that serve you in school, career, and family. Sports also has its dangers, physical and emotional. This book helps you seize the opportunities of sports, and shun the dangers. That's our only agenda. Our Web site, A-Game.com, continues the story with updates, interviews, and a community forum. We're not out to get you to play at a particular college, use a particular product, or wear a particular shoe. We provide a safe harbor, full of objective information. We give you the tools to make sports a positive experience, and, perhaps most important, to keep it all in perspective.

How to Use This Book

In these pages you'll find dozens of ways to get the edge in sports, school, and life. Read the whole book to get the big picture. Read it with pen or highlighter in hand to mark the key things to do right now, at this point in your journey. Become familiar with the book and you'll refer to it as new situations arise.

The earlier in your life you read *The Student-Athlete Survival Guide,* the better. But the information is useful whether you are a high school or college athlete, whether you are a "blue-chip" recruit or an average player, whether you play basketball or football or compete in a non-revenue-producing sport. And whether you are male or female.

We encourage you to share this book with key adults in your life. In appendix 1 there's even a special message for parents or others you look to for advice.

Chapter 8, on athletic scholarships and other forms of financial aid, advises you to make "apples-to-apples" comparisons of financial aid packages from different colleges. The chapter even provides a formula for doing so. You could calculate it with pencil and paper, and keep the results in a file folder or notebook. Or, go to our Web site and plug the numbers into our online financial-aid calculator. (You may want to ask your parents to help.) By doing that you create documents you can print and save to your hard drive for future reference. Read *The Guide* and visit A-Game.com to play the game of your life.

Find Your Own Answers

When we speak to groups of athletes, we usually start by asking two important questions: why do you play sports, and what do you hope to gain from sports?

Athletes constantly tell us how useful those questions are. You can be so busy playing your sport that you don't think about why you're doing it. Once you stop to think it over, you're on your way to maximizing the enjoyment and reward of sports.

A high school athlete once told us that one of the main reasons she plays basketball is the attention she gets as the starting point guard on a top-ranked team. Her goal, she said, was to play in college. But the minute she came up with those answers, she saw some problems.

This athlete was spending so much time enjoying her popularity that she wasn't working enough to improve her game or lead her team. Her early success was based on natural athletic ability. Now, players who were working harder were catching up to her. She was also coasting in the classroom. In her junior year, although the work was getting harder, she wasn't studying harder. Her grades were slipping—and that would hurt her chances of getting into her number-one college choice.

Take a moment and write down your answers to those two key questions: why do you play sports, and what do you hope to gain from sports? By focusing on why you play and what you hope to accomplish, you will take a step toward achieving your goals. You'll gain the edge, for 90 percent of the people you compete against don't think about their objectives or make a plan to reach them. They often look for shortcuts. But there are no shortcuts to genuine success, and the people who seek them out end up cheating themselves.

Why Should You Read This Book?

By answering the questions above, you've discovered one reason why you should read this book. *The Student-Athlete Survival Guide* helps you identify your goals. The next step is to ask yourself how you can reach them.

Experience is the best teacher. In this book, you'll gain access to the experience of hundreds of athletes who have dealt with situations similar to yours.

You'll also read messages from people who are legends in the world of sport, such as NFL Hall of Fame member Ronnie Lott (see Pregame, page x); Basketball Hall of Fame member Ann Meyers Drysdale (see Halftime, page 85); and Mike Krzyzewski, head basketball coach at Duke University (see Postgame, page 157). We also draw on our own experiences, and we've each added a personal note at the end of this chapter.

Making mistakes is a great way to learn, and sometimes you just have to make your own. But why not learn from the mistakes (and correct decisions) of others? It's a lot less painful.

Playing and *competing* are synonyms when it comes to athletics. A lot of the enjoyment and satisfaction in sports comes from constantly trying to improve and trying to win. This book shows you how to get the most out of your commitment.

Male or Female, Athletes Are Athletes

Whether you are male or female, there is no better training ground for life than sports. Buzzwords that are synonymous with success in corporate America originated in the sports world: teamwork, leadership, goal setting, determination. Participating in sports has long-term rewards that can last well beyond your years as a competitor. It can prepare you for career success and help you start a lifelong habit of working out to maintain your health and well-being.

We thankfully live in an era where it's cool for females to play sports. We could quote statistics to prove that girls who participate in athletics have higher self-esteem, are more likely to stay in school, and are less likely to get pregnant or use alcohol or other drugs. And you know that those women soaring over hurdles or running a fast break on the basketball court are not the ones trying to prove their maturity by sucking on cigarettes. Statistics aside, there is one driving truth: participating in sports is more fun, far more exciting, and more rewarding than hanging out at the mall.

A federal law, Title IX, mandates gender equity in sports. One example of how this law mandates equality is in how athletic scholarships are administered: the number of athletic scholarships awarded to women must reflect the percentage of females in the general student population of the school.

Many people are under the impression that Title IX only recently became law, but in fact this mandate has been in effect since 1972. However, it has taken time to bring about equality. For example, the NCAA and its member colleges did not comply for a couple of decades, and it took several bangs on the head from the Federal courts and threats by Congress to withhold funds. Finally, the sports world is wide open for females. Of the 796 teams added by NCAA schools in 1998–99, 515 are women's. To achieve gender equity, many colleges are actively recruiting women for athletic scholarships.

The fight for equality in women's sports, however, is not over. Some colleges have complied with the legal requirements rather than the spirit of Title IX by eliminating men's teams instead of adding women's teams. Men's gymnastics, volleyball, tennis, and in some cases even football teams have been the victims.

Title IX's effect on the sports world did not happen by itself. Hundreds of women who excelled at athletics became living illustrations of excellence in sport. Notable personalities such as tennis star Martina Navratilova and track great Jackie Joyner-Kersee have brought women's sports into the limelight. And success stories in the headlines continue to bring more attention to women's sports. In the 1996 Olympics, the U.S. softball team's gold-medal performance put the spotlight on women in sports. The U.S. soccer team's phenomenal victory in the 1999 Women's World Cup showcased women's athletics in America as never before—and this event continues to be a springboard for greater exposure and wider opportunity in athletics for women.

The work toward equality may not be over, but it's a great time to be a female athlete!

Been There: A Word from Marc Isenberg

Our goal with this book is to give you information that will help you thrive in sports and school. And not after the fact! The less you have to say, "I wish I'd known then what I know now," the better off you will be.

This book is about being proactive. When I was a kid, my grandfather used to tell me, "You don't know what you don't know." As a former know-it-all, this was hard advice to swallow, and I didn't follow his wisdom as much as I should have. I know now that there are times in your life when you just have to trust that you don't have all the answers. Despite how stubborn most of us are (especially headstrong athletes), you can benefit greatly from the wisdom of people who know how the game is played.

When it comes to balancing athletics and academics, I learned the hard way. I was forced off the Emory University basketball team when the coach saw that I was not living up to my potential in the classroom. I regret that my college basketball career ended this way, but I'm grateful to Coach Lloyd Winston for his wake-up call.

I earned a degree in finance at Emory, but my real education was in playing, reading, and following sports. Many of my study sessions in the library were spent reading back issues of *Sports Illustrated,* and my real major was the business of college athletics.

Looking back at age 32, I know I learned from my mistakes. I didn't get college credit for what I spent most of my time doing. But my education and the time I spent at Emory enabled me to pursue my interests and write this book. To do this, I teamed up with Rick Rhoads, who is not only a great wordsmith but a person with an older and much wiser perspective.

It's a Great Life If You Don't Weaken: A Word from Rick Rhoads

My dad Lester (everyone, including me, called him Lester) was a college professor who also operated a summer camp in Maine that specialized in sailing. As a teenager, I raced sailboats. When my regular crew members went home at the end of the summer, Lester would crew for me. He was a sailor, but he didn't know much about racing.

After leading for most of one race, several boats suddenly passed us. We'd been winning more than our share of races, and I'd become arrogant about leading the series. Suddenly I turned from a cool yachtsman to a baffled 14-year-old boy feeling humiliated in front of his father. I kicked the cockpit rail and said some bad words about the impossibility of the other boats catching us so fast.

Lester calmly asked, "Rick, what do you think we're doing wrong?" I realized that instead of looking for a solution, I was making a fool of myself. Lester didn't know the answer, but he was expressing confidence in me to find it.

I did figure out the problem, which hardly matters now. But the real lesson I learned was to take a mature approach to adversity. That lesson helped me through many problems in sports and in school— and in being a father, which is the perspective I bring to these pages.

As a parent, I've participated in the college and graduate school selection process, and I have been called on for advice in career decisions. Raising kids (and being raised by them) has been a rough but rewarding voyage—especially rough during the teenage years. My wife Peggy had an eye on the big picture, and she helped me survive.

So did laughter. Life can be serious and funny. During the hundreds of hours Marc and I spent together writing this book, we laughed so loudly that my wife would ask, "Are you working?" We laughed mostly about things that happen in sports, about crazy things and even about horrible things—like the father of a football player who sharpened the buckle on his son's helmet to cut opponents. Laughing beat crying.

We've edited and rewritten this book many times, in an effort to make it clear and useful. Let us know what you think of this guide and what you get out of it. You'll help improve the next edition for the athletes who come after you.

This book outlines everything you need to do to succeed in high school, to select the right college for you, and to succeed at college. Doing well in college will give you a running start toward achieving success for the rest of your life—the years, hopefully 60, 70, or 80 of them, after your college graduation.

CHAPTER 2

The Ingredients of Success

A lot of effort goes into being successful. In high school, you have to balance sports, academics, social life, responsibilities at home, and maybe a part-time job. You need to take the right courses and prepare for college entrance exams. You need to select the right college, which can be complicated, particularly when the pressures of recruiting come into play.

Once you're at college, the demands of athletics and academics become even greater, but you still have to balance them. As a college student, you have to select the right major and plan your next step—whether that's going on to graduate school or starting a career. Even your social life gets more serious as you find lifelong friends and maybe even a spouse.

Doing all of this well sounds hard, but life is a juggling act. If you're not feeling the pressure, check your pulse. Just pay attention to the details and understand how each detail helps you achieve your goals. Once you do that, you can succeed and enjoy the process.

One accomplishment leads to the next, and after a while success becomes habit forming. Remember that lots of people—many of whom are no smarter than you are—have succeeded, so you know it can't be all that hard. Success is doable and enjoyable, particularly when you make good friends along the way.

But there are many ways to fail in our society. Plenty of people find them. You can probably spot classmates who are on their way.

If you read this book from a different angle, it provides detailed directions on how to fail. Just do everything the book says not to do and we guarantee you will fail! But if you'd rather succeed, here are the key ingredients you'll need.

Passion

When you were a little kid on a trip with your family, did you drive your parents crazy by asking, "Are we there yet?"

What's wrong with that question? It makes the destination the reward. Successful people agree that the journey is the reward. They love what they are doing, even when they are struggling to reach their goal. The harder the road, the sweeter it is when they get to their destination.

If you want to find lasting success, find something you're passionate about—something you enjoy doing, thinking about, and talking about. Make it a goal that captures your imagination—a journey that, like a good story, you don't want to end.

Balance

Passion leads to success, but unlimited passion can get out of control and mess you up. That's where balance comes in.

For example, let's say that your passion is to become financially secure and to have all the opportunities you never had growing up. You work hard and you make $10 million. But along the way you mistreat everybody around you. You may end up a rich person, but you are surrounded by enemies. Would that be success?

Balance means paying attention to all the important things in your life. It also means keeping an eye on the future as well as the present.

You might feel happiest now when you play ball or run or swim. And reading books (except, of course, this one) or sitting in a classroom doesn't make you happy at all. But do you think the same things that make you happy now will make you happy in five, ten, or twenty years? Will playing your sport night and day get you a good job and a comfortable home? If not, shouldn't you do what you enjoy now while also working hard at the things that seem difficult or boring but are necessary for your future happiness?

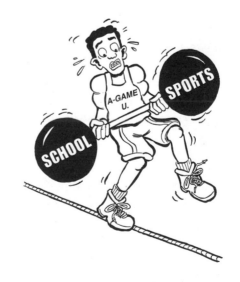

Don't be afraid to tackle the tough tasks: when you tackle challenging tasks, especially those you think you're not capable of, you may surprise yourself with your own ability and the sense of pride and satisfaction you feel.

Perspective

As great as sports are, we shouldn't lose sight of the fact that, in the grand scheme of things, sports are a pretty small part of life.

If you're a young athlete living in an ESPN world, it might be difficult to comprehend this. However, ask someone who has experienced the death of a loved one just how important the state finals are. They may help you gain some perspective. It's fine to get caught up in the excitement of sports, but it's also important to understand that a big part of life lies outside of athletics.

Apart from that, it's necessary for you to realize that there is life *after* sports. What are your priorities in life? Do you live only for the moment, or are you also thinking about the future? Do you realize that when you're done playing competitive sports, there are decades of life to live?

Consistent Hard Work

"The harder I work, the luckier I get." That's a statement you might hear often. Those with the discipline to work hard over a long period of time are ready to take advantage of a break when it comes along. Your smarts, talent, personality, and good looks will take you a certain distance. But as you grow up, you enter the competitive world. Without putting in the necessary effort, you don't stand a chance against those who develop the habit of hard work.

We've all seen cases where an athlete had so much talent that she excelled without trying. But suddenly, the others catch up, and that natural athlete gets frustrated when she is no longer the star. The same thing happens to some students who find it easy to get good grades: they never develop the study habits necessary for success in the long run.

Work often gets a bad rap in our society. Try an experiment. Ask people of any age what they like to do. We predict that most will reply with something from this list: "Go to the beach, go skiing, listen to music, play ball, go shopping, hang out, watch TV, travel, dance, see a movie." A few will say they like to read. Hardly any will say they like to work or study.

But if you are doing the work necessary to turn your dreams into reality, why not enjoy it? That's more satisfying than lying on the beach.

The beach is enjoyable as a break from hard work. It's the icing on the cake, not the cake itself.

Preparation

The ability to think ahead is key to success. One of the greatest teachers of all time, Coach John Wooden, who led UCLA to ten NCAA men's basketball championships in twelve years, said it very simply: "Failing to prepare is preparing to fail."

Suppose a college you are interested in requires you to take advanced algebra. You know you can take the course next year, but you don't bother looking into the details right now.

The deadline for setting up your classes for your senior year comes. You go to enroll in advanced algebra, but there is one problem: you needed to take a more basic course in your junior year to be eligible for the advanced algebra class. Now, you can't get into the class and you're missing a key requirement for applying to the college of your choice. Planning reduces such unpleasant surprises.

Maturity

As we grow and learn more, we see how big the world is, how infinite the knowledge, and just how little of it each of us really grasps. Therefore, we should become more open to advice, suggestions, and help from others. Of course, as we gain experience, we should evaluate all advice critically, even when it comes from people we trust and hold in high esteem. There's a joke that college freshmen think they know everything about a subject after reading one book about it. Then they read another book, which contradicts the first book, and suddenly they know much less than they thought. But it's no joke that know-it-alls rarely succeed. Even those who do well for a while get left behind when life moves on and they are unable to grasp new developments. Truly mature people remain open to learning and improving even as they become clearer and more certain about what they know and do.

Initiative

There's a big difference between being obedient and taking initiative. If it's your job to take out the garbage and you do it when you're told, that's obedience. If you see that the garbage container is full and you take it out without being asked, that's initiative.

Initiative is closely tied to maturity. Nobody expects a two-year-old to be a self-starter (except in tearing up the place). As you get older, success requires doing what the situation requires and not waiting for your parents, teachers, or coaches to spell out every detail. Initiative also requires finding out what is required for success.

Suppose you miss a class because of a road trip. Would you find out what took place in that class, including any assignments that were given out, or would you simply wait for the ax to fall? We trust you know which choice the person who takes initiative would make!

Seeing the Big Picture

There is no rule that says life will always give you what you want. Sometimes you have to do certain things, not because you want to but because those things are stepping-stones to your goals.

For example, you might choose a school where you won't play much as a freshman. However, that school has a strong team and an excellent coach, and you'll get good training that will serve you better in the long run. Or you might have to choose between two jobs, and one pays less than the other. You might want the extra money, but you might choose the job that pays less because it will give you better training and experience for the future.

Whatever your goal, long-term success requires attention to the stepping-stones that don't necessarily give you immediate payoffs.

Looking beyond athletics is important, too: when you focus only on your sport, you miss the big picture. When your athletic career is over you want to be ready to go on to other successes. It's fine to pursue a dream; but putting all your hopes on making it big in professional sports is like staking your future on winning the lottery.

No matter how talented you are, you're never more than an injury away from the end of your athletic career. Your plan should prepare you for success—no matter how far you go as an athlete. If you remain ignorant about the world around you, you set yourself up for a fall. That's happened to many professional athletes who were once rich and famous, and then just famous. Their money disappeared and reappeared in the hands of others.

Ignorance allows you to be taken advantage of. By educating yourself you earn the respect of others. It's similar to what happens when you're part of a team. You want respect from your teammates, so you work hard to prepare for your role.

What really motivates us? It's not only money. Sometimes money is just the way we keep score. We want other people to accept us, to value our ideas and opinions. Above all to respect us.

Values

Your list of things to do might sound like this: get to practice; get ready for a math midterm; write an English paper; get to your part-time job; watch your little brother. Sometimes you have to run fast just to stay in the same place, let alone advance!

But what happens to the things that are most important to you in the meantime? Your relationships with family and friends? Your ethical or religious beliefs? Your concerns about society? When you are constantly rushing around, it's easy to lose track of your basic values and it's tempting to take shortcuts.

Maybe you accept a good grade without doing the work. Or drugs are going around at a party, everyone seems to be enjoying them, and you join in.

A shortcut will always get you somewhere—but it's rarely where you want to go. All of us need to step back every so often and ask ourselves, "What's it all about? What kind of a person do I want to be? What should I be thinking about when I make decisions?" When you are young and changing fast, these are critical questions. One way or the other, you will become an adult. You can pay attention to how you grow and develop—or just let it happen any old way. Why not direct your own production?

These big issues are tough to deal with. In appendix 2, we give you a set of questions to think about grouped by topic (see page 164). Only one of the topic areas is about sports. You might think the other parts are unimportant, and if we tell you that athletics should not be your number-one priority at this time in your life, you might reply, "Are you kidding?" But keep in mind that throughout your life, your priorities will change. Ten years from now you may have a spouse and children. You don't want to regret that you never made an effort to be productive outside of sports.

Friends You Can Count On

It's a dog-eat-dog world. Who can you trust? On the other hand, if you never learn which friend you can trust, you'll never find people you can count on. And how can anybody be successful without a few close friends? You share your thoughts, goals, and fears with friends. Friends help you understand the world and even yourself.

To a large degree, your success or failure is determined by the people you surround yourself with. The wrong friends drag you down. Peer pressure is on all those lists of reasons why people get drunk or take drugs. Should you select friends who encourage you to practice and study, or who champion the joys of ditching school? Should you have friends who help you figure out how to succeed, or tell you why you can't? The right kinds of friends lift you up, like a point guard who raises everybody's level of play.

Of course, there will be times when even the right friends make bad decisions. That's when your independent judgment and self-confidence will see you through.

You're going to spend a lot of time in high school and college with your teammates, and some of them will naturally become close friends. But you might have to go out of your way to make a close friend who doesn't participate in organized sports. It's worth the effort: you need a friend who has a different viewpoint.

And Finally, a Sense of Humor

If you never crack a smile, you can depress yourself and those around you. Remember that even grim situations have their funny side.

If someone disrespects you, is it best to brood about it, fight about it, or laugh it off? It depends on the situation, but laughter is often the best way to put the incident in its proper perspective.

People with well-developed senses of humor can laugh at themselves. In the Pregame, Ronnie Lott talks about learning from mistakes (page x). That's really the main way we learn anything. Changing and learning new skills is often difficult. It can be frustrating, depressing, and, sometimes—worst of all—embarrassing. But if you can pick yourself out of the mud and laugh about it, rather than wallow in your own misfortune, you can help yourself recover and advance. And people will like you for it.

So take life seriously. And lighten up!

CHAPTER 3

Roadblocks to Success

As every student knows, cheating is rampant in our high schools and colleges. At one university over half of the MBA students in a class were caught cheating on a test. The subject of the course? Business ethics. Plagiarism is more widespread than ever, partly as a result of easy access to material on the Internet. In sports, some coaches cheat—for example, by violating recruiting rules. And some athletes cheat—for example, by using banned substances such as steroids.

Why is cheating so prevalent? There is tremendous pressure to succeed and win, to beat the competition. That should inspire everybody to work hard rather than cheat. But we live in a microwave society. Insert the food, push the button, and—ding!—24 seconds later, instant gratification. Even if they haven't prepared for a test, many students still want to find a way to get an A.

So many students cheat that they put peer pressure on those who don't cheat or cooperate with cheaters. The mentality is that everybody's doing it, so it must be all right. Sports talk show host Jim Rome mocks the widespread acceptance of cheating in sports by saying, "If you're not cheating, you're not trying."

The Just Rewards of Cheating

A high school sophomore facing a situation where his grades could threaten his eligibility to play sports rationalizes cheating this way. "If I don't get a B on this book report, my average in English will be too low and Mr. Dempsey—that sports-hating creep—will turn me in to the coach. But I haven't read the book and now there's no time. I'll get Geoffrey to write my report. He's cool for a nerd. I let him hang around with me and the other guys on the team. Geoff is clever. He'll write a paper good enough so Dempsey will believe I worked hard. But he'll make enough mistakes so Dempsey won't suspect anything, and I'll be able to play Saturday."

If this sophomore believes that the only reason not to cheat is the risk of getting caught, his analysis makes sense. Ineligibility would hurt, so why not avoid it? After all, you're punished only when you get caught. And most of the time, you don't get caught.

But is it true that cheaters are punished only when they are caught? Read on.

How to Get Good Grades and Fail

Imagine this scenario. You are flunking a course, but you are the high school phenom and there's pressure on your teacher or an administrator to change your grade or to find someone to do your work for you. Some teachers won't go along with this; others allow themselves to be pressured into it; some get caught up in the excitement and lose sight of their responsibilities as educators.

The question is, do you help yourself by accepting this kind of "aid"? Keeping your eligibility this way may help a coach's career. It may result in more wins, so that the community is happy. But what does it do for you? It makes you eligible but dumb. It teaches you to look for the easy way out, a habit that is guaranteed to lead you to trouble. This kind of aid is far worse for you than money and gifts from people with their own agendas. Those can cost you your athletic eligibility, but faking grades can cost you your ability to think.

If you were this athlete, your own mental calculations should go more like this. "If I don't do my own schoolwork, I will not learn how to read, write, or do math well. In fact, I won't really know how to reason clearly—at least not if it requires seeing beyond the obvious. Even if I do become a pro, do I want to be a know-nothing fool?

"Furthermore, once I start down the cheating track, it will become a vicious cycle. My whole life will be about taking shortcuts, looking for the easy way out. Even if I know I won't get caught, even if the people around me are helping me cheat, I've got to check myself because it's wrong. And ultimately it will mess up my life and the lives of my family and friends."

As University of Massachusetts (UMass) basketball player Jameel Pugh puts it, "Some people say you need an education to fall back on in case you don't make it. That's true. But if you do make it to the NBA, you need an education to deal with the business aspects and also to protect yourself from the many questionable characters that money seems to attract."

Nobody Said Cheaters Are Smart

Some athletes cheat so obviously that they contribute to the dumb jock myth. A group of college football players were caught with illegally obtained handicapped parking permits. How could they have believed that nobody would notice a bunch of the biggest and strongest guys on campus leaping out of their cars and striding off to their destinations?

This was probably not the first time these athletes had taken short-cuts. There are many people who actively help athletes "beat the system." Some look the other way; some do it because they really think they are helping; most have their own agendas. To be a successful athlete requires confidence. That's a good quality when it's backed by talent and experience. But confidence can turn into cockiness. And a cocky athlete believes he'll succeed in an area where he does not have the skill or smarts to justify that belief.

Character Counts

Supermodel Jerry Hall said, "If I weren't so beautiful, maybe I'd have more character." This is an insightful comment from a person who receives special treatment because of a particular talent or gift. But where will she be once age leaves her unable to meet the conventional standards of beauty? Unfortunately, there are many athletes who could say, "If I weren't so talented, maybe I'd have more character." Where will they be once the cheering stops?

As Pogo says, "We have seen the enemy, and it is us!" Don't justify cheating by saying, "Well, everybody else does it." If the next guy is cheating to gain an advantage, work harder so you can win without cheating. That goes for academics and sports. It's not as easy in the short run, but you end up better, stronger, and smarter. Keep in mind that sports is training for life in general. Your athletic career will not be the only high point of your life: it's a springboard to further success.

Sportsmanship Counts

When former Chicago Bear great Walter Payton scored a touchdown, he just handed the ball to the official. When asked why he didn't celebrate by spiking the ball (crazy rituals were not yet in vogue), he answered, "I want to act like I've been there before." Athletes are often told that it's important to demonstrate good sportsmanship because they represent something bigger than themselves: their school or the traditions of their sport. That's true, but a bad sport hurts himself as well. The way you treat other people tells a lot about how you value yourself. If an athlete tries to win by intentionally injuring an opponent, that athlete is saying, "I'm not good enough to win if I play by the rules." Or if he shows up an opponent, he's saying, "I can only look good by making you look bad."

How to Destroy Yourself

In today's society there is a range of ways you can harm or even kill yourself, including drugs, booze, tobacco, crime, unsafe sex, and reckless driving. Sometimes people harm themselves or take foolish risks because they feel overwhelmed. It can be hard to talk to friends and family about what troubles you, but try to do it. Your problems will usually look less overwhelming and easier to deal with. If you think it will help or don't know where else to turn, talk with a professional counselor.

Athletes are subject to all of the above dangers, and there are more too. There are pressures to become bigger, faster, stronger—whatever it takes, whatever the risks. The pressure can come from all directions: from athletes themselves, coaches, and even parents who want their children to excel in sports at all costs.

Steroids, Creatine, and Andro

Many athletes have used steroids to become stronger and faster. You shouldn't. Steroids can cause severe mental and physical diseases; in some cases, they even lead to death. Every organization that governs sports—from the International Olympic Committee (IOC) to the NCAA—bans athletes who test positive for steroids. But the Drug Enforcement Agency reports that despite these bans, the percentage of high school students who have used steroids has increased over 50 percent in the past four years, from 1.8 percent to 2.8 percent.

In the 1990s, a muscle-building supplement called *creatine* became popular with athletes. Some doctors believe creatine may harm the kidneys and other organs, or even cause emotional changes. Studies done so far are inconclusive. No one knows the long-term effects of creatine, just as no one in the 1950s knew the long-term effects of smoking cigarettes.

A professional athlete who happens to be very strong and breaks home-run records took androstenedione (andro)—a substance that is legal (as we write) in Major League Baseball but banned by the NCAA, the National Football League (NFL), and IOC. Does this mean you should run out to your local drugstore and start using andro? Or is it significant that Mark McGwire stopped using this substance?

There's nothing wrong with looking for whatever advantage you can. As long as it's legal and, more importantly, is proven not to be harmful. But that's the problem.

The label on Andro-6 contains this caution: "Because of the potency of this formula, Andro-6 should not be used by women, anyone under 18 years of age, or people suffering from any medical conditions, including, but not limited to, diabetes, heart disease, psychological disorders and prostate hypertrophy."

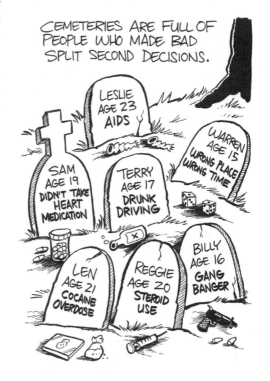

AndroGel, available by prescription, is touted by its manufacturer as an "easy-to-apply testosterone ointment" to treat male testosterone deficiency. The buzz in the sports community is that it will become the newest craze because it's an innocent-seeming ointment rather than a scary injection. Testosterone can boost muscle mass and sexual drive, and it can cause liver damage and exacerbate prostate cancer.

Creatine and andro are available without prescription, over the counter. They are considered nutritional supplements and are not regulated by the Food and Drug Administration. Unlike pharmaceutical products, nutritional supplements carry no requirements for animal and human research studies before they are made available to the public. And because they are not classified as foods, they are not even subject to food labeling laws. So the bottom line is, you don't really know what's in the bottle. One athlete failed a drug test after taking a product labeled Chinese Herbal Medicine. The product contained steroids.

Rather than taking supplements, ask yourself if you're doing everything you can to improve your strength and quickness. There are no shortcuts to success in sports. The answer isn't a pill or powder: it's a lot of hard work.

There is no doubt that other magic potions are on their way to the locker room. We urge you to avoid unproven and potentially dangerous substances—even if they are not banned. Don't risk your health, your sanity, or your life for a marginal advantage.

Athletes and Crime

In these times, it's hard to distinguish the sports pages from the police blotter. There are hundreds of talk show hosts, journalists, and psychologists who tell us why so many athletes break rules and commit crimes. It really doesn't matter why. (In fact, people in all walks of life commit crimes, but it's more spectacular news when an athlete ruins a promising career by doing so.) All that matters from your standpoint is that you learn how to tell right from wrong and you learn how to stay out of trouble.

It's really not that hard. There's a famous saying: "The best defense against the bomb is not to be there when it goes off." It's the same with avoiding trouble. Don't get yourself in situations where trouble is likely to occur. And if you find yourself where trouble is about to happen, get yourself out of that situation, quickly!

One athlete who was insulted by a belligerent drunk said, "I had no choice but to retaliate, because he tested my manhood." Grow up. You need to keep your cool even if the person deserves to be punched in the mouth. It's not worth risking your career. You might be convicted of assault (think jail time), and you don't know who you are dealing with. That person can pull a gun out and shoot you. Cemeteries are full of people who made bad split-second decisions.

CHAPTER 4

Get the Edge in Sports

In the sports world, there is a lot of talk about *getting the edge*. It means becoming a better athlete and a better competitor. But how do you do that?

Hall of Famer Satchell Paige may have been the greatest pitcher of all time. He played in the Negro Leagues for twenty-two years, and he often dominated Major League hitters in exhibition games. In 1948, after Major League Baseball finally allowed African Americans in, he joined the Cleveland Indians and played in the Majors for six years, until he was into his fifties.

Satchell Paige is known for his pithy sayings. The most famous is, "Don't look back. Something might be gaining on you." This is profound advice if you want to get the edge in sports. If you shouldn't look back, where should you look? Look ahead!

Plot Your Future

As an athlete, you've learned the value of preparation.

Preparation begins with a plan. To succeed, you have to practice a lot—but you have to be smart about how you practice. You have to know which skills to work on now and which to focus on later. You have to know what kind of strength training and conditioning your sport requires. You have to visualize where you want to be—in a week, a month, a year, and several years from now. Then you need to make an overall plan about how to get there and break the plan down into steps you can achieve each day.

Preparation puts you in position to compete with confidence. When the starting gun goes off or the first pitch comes, you'll know you are as ready as you can be. You'll have the mental edge to play your best: win or lose, you'll go home feeling positive about your performance and you'll be ready to do better next time.

Think Like Mike

You can practice shooting eight hours a day, but if your technique is wrong, then all you get is very good at shooting the wrong way. Get the fundamentals down and the level of everything you do will rise.

—Michael Jordan

One of Michael Jordan's great strengths was his ability to work on his weaknesses. In college basketball, his athleticism allowed him to blow by defenders. So they played off him—which they could get away with because of his mediocre jump shot. Michael responded by spending hours working to improve his jumper.

When Michael came into the NBA, he was 6 foot, 6 inches and 195 pounds. Defenders countered his moves and his jump shot by pushing him around. So Michael responded again, by putting in hours in the weight room with a tough regimen that he continued throughout his career.

The additional 20 pounds of muscle he built made him impossible to defend without double-teaming. He responded again and did daily dribble and quickness drills, which is something many NBA players haven't bothered with since high school (if then).

Michael's Work Ethic

In his book *Loose Balls,* New Jersey Nets power forward Jayson Williams writes that as much as Michael Jordan was acclaimed, he was underrated. Everyone saw MJ's ability, but few understood his effect on his teammates and on his opponents.

Michael set an example by working on every part of his game, from dribbling and passing to foul shots and defense. He was in the gym early, and he left late. He played with the same intensity level at practice as he did in a championship game with millions of people watching. He demanded that others do the same, leading his team to higher levels of play. Michael intimidated his opponents. They knew that whether they had to play offense or defense against him, they had better be ready for a war: Michael always brought his A-game. As Michael's legend continues to build, we're beginning to realize he was a once-in-a-millennium athlete.

You and Michael

Maybe you can't "Be like Mike" in the sense of being the greatest player in your sport, but you can give the same effort. Set goals. As Michael said, "You have to expect things of yourself before you can do them." Figure out every step you need to take to reach your goals, then make a plan. If you pay attention to the details, work hard even when progress is not visible, and think and act like Mike, there is no question that you will make the most of your potential.

Take the Controls

Your sport is filled with variables: the wind, the officiating, illness, injury, your opponents. These are variables that are not under your control. To get the edge, focus on the things you can control.

Let's take a look at the key areas that are largely under your control. In addition to your sport-specific fundamentals, the elements you can control are nutrition, rest, fitness, and sports psychology. If you want to delve deeper into any of these topics, there are many books, videos, and Web sites available (see appendix 3, Resources). You can also consult qualified specialists in these areas.

"You Are What You Eat"

That adage may not be entirely true, but it contains an element of truth. Eat the foods that give you the right nutrition and you'll have the energy to play your best and grow stronger and faster.

Many people know that, but what do they actually do? They consume burgers, fries, shakes, and donuts—regardless of the amount of fat they contain. Some seek quick energy from sweets, only to feel listless two hours later. Others obsess about their diets and follow one fad after another.

The one-sided, extreme diets don't work in the long run—which is why there's always a market for nutty diet books by diet gurus, diet videos, and weight-loss and weight-gain programs. And just as plentiful as all these diet products are convenience stores and fast food restaurants with trillions of pounds of junk food. Take a look the next time you're at the checkout counter: you can fill your shopping cart full of Twinkies and then pick up a dozen magazines on diet and nutrition!

What's the best approach to nutrition? Ask any doctor or nutritionist who isn't involved in the billion-dollar diet bonanza and they'll likely refer you to the Food Guide Pyramid developed by the U.S. Department of Agriculture (USDA).

This pyramid, which is part of the USDA's Dietary Guidelines for Americans, illustrates the recommended number of daily servings you should eat from five of the six basic food groups. The base of the pyramid (the widest part) shows you the foods that should comprise the main part of your diet. As you ascend the pyramid, the sections get narrower and represent foods that are good for you but that you should eat in smaller quantities. The USDA notes that some foods fit into more than one group. For example, dry beans, peas, and lentils can be counted as daily servings in either the meat-and-beans group or the vegetable group. A list of what constitutes a serving in each food group is noted below.

WHAT COUNTS AS A SERVING?

Bread, Cereal, Rice, and Pasta
1 slice of bread
1 ounce of ready-to-eat cereal
½ cup of cooked cereal, rice, or pasta

Vegetable
1 cup of raw leafy vegetables
½ cup of other vegetables—cooked or chopped raw
¾ cup of vegetable juice

Fruit
1 medium apple, banana, or orange
½ cup of chopped, cooked, or canned fruit
¾ cup of vegetable juice

Milk, Yogurt, and Cheese
1 cup of milk or yogurt
1½ ounces of natural cheese
2 ounces of processed cheese

Meat, Poultry, Fish, Dry Beans, Eggs, and Nuts
2–3 ounces of cooked lean meat, poultry, or fish

½ cup of cooked dry beans or 1 egg counts as 1 ounce of lean meat

2 tablespoons of peanut butter or ⅓ cup of nuts count as 1 ounce of meat

The Food Guide Pyramid is the best nutritional guide ever created, but it hasn't had a publicity machine behind it—no appearances on talk show circuits, no recommendations by Oprah. There's nothing to sell: it's free! Just add water. It's important for your body's metabolism to consume about eight glasses of water or the equivalent (sports drinks, juice) each day. Drink even more if you are working out and sweating.

How much should you eat? The answer is simple. If you are getting too thin, eat more. If you are gaining excessive body fat, eat less. Your weight naturally fluctuates a pound or two from day to day. Decide how much to eat based on changes over a period of several weeks or months.

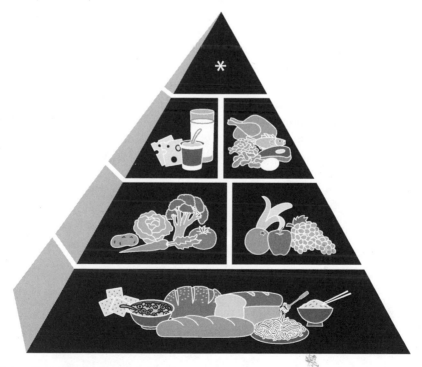

*Fats, oils, and sweets: eat sparingly.

Source: The Food Guide Pyramid, Home and Garden Bulletin No. 252, Center for Nutrition Policy and Promotion, U.S. Department of Agriculture, Oct. 1996

Body Image

Look at the "beautiful people" in the movies, on TV, and in ads. They supposedly define the ideal way to look. This causes many people to go through unnecessary grief, because most of us don't look quite like that. For example, how many women are as thin as some of the stars of TV shows and movies? In fact, why should they want to be? Often, the bodies on the screen are the result of anorexia, bulimia, and a surgeon's knife.

A similar dynamic occurs in sports. Football linemen are supposed to be huge, so some guys do whatever it takes to bulk up, including pigging out on high-fat, high-calorie foods. Female gymnasts are supposed to look like prepubescent girls, so some athletes starve themselves to prevent natural development from taking place. Some wrestlers also starve themselves to "make weight."

What's wrong with this? Eating too much fat or sugar can increase the chances of developing heart disease, cancer, diabetes, and many other life-threatening disorders. Not eating enough nutrients can lead to liver and kidney failure and threaten the central nervous system. By trying to alter your body's natural metabolism and growth, you can trade short-term gain for long-term risk.

Sometimes the risk materializes all too soon. In December 1997, University of Michigan wrestler Jeff Reese tried to lose 21 pounds in four days so that he could qualify for the 150-pound weight class. After a four-hour weight-loss session in a 92° F room, Jeff died. At around the same time, three other college wrestlers around the United States died while trying to make weight.

It's fine to eat and exercise to get bigger and stronger. If you're trying to stay light, you should certainly avoid overeating. But avoid extreme and dangerous measures, even if they are recommended by a coach or parent. If you are not sure, consult an objective expert.

Your Health Bank

A balanced diet provides an even supply of energy. That's what athletes need to consistently practice and compete at the highest possible level. Eating right is like putting money in the bank, so that it will be there for your future. In this case, you're helping to guarantee your body's future.

Rest for the Weary

Some people have trouble sleeping. Most athletes are lucky in this respect, because when you work out regularly, it's easier to fall asleep. The challenge is usually to stay awake and get your schoolwork done. For peak athletic performance, it's important to get enough rest. As much as possible, establish a regular time to go to bed and to wake up—and stick to it. Consistent, adequate rest allows you to play hard, concentrate, and focus. If you are tired, you risk injury, because your body does not respond the way you think it will.

Survival of the Fittest

With the right approach, athletes can push themselves to amazing levels of accomplishment. (Just think about what it takes to run a marathon.) Whatever your sport, your performance depends on your muscular strength, flexibility, and endurance, which is largely a function of how well your cardiovascular system functions. Therefore, physical conditioning is a key aspect of getting the edge.

How do you get into the best possible shape? It's similar to nutrition: too much training or too little training is bad. Like Goldilocks, you want it to be "just right." For athletes, that means working your butt off without getting run down or injured.

You won't see progress every day, but don't be discouraged. In real life, progress comes in jumps. The rest of the time, you're on a plateau or you may even take a few steps back.

The Smart (and Short) Guide to Fitness

Here are some fitness guidelines to follow.

- **Stretch and warm up before and after you lift, practice, or compete.** Stretching improves your performance by making you more flexible, and it reduces the chances of injury while training or playing. For stretching to work, you have to do it properly. Your coach or trainer will have stretching routines. Effective stretching involves holding the stretched position for 15 seconds or more.

  Lifting free weights (or your own body weight) or using exercise machines to the point of muscle failure (inability to do another repetition) are the most effective methods of building maximum strength. But they also contain the potential for injury.

Minimize the chance of injury by stretching, using the right equipment, using good form, resting sufficiently between sessions, and alternating muscle groups.

Athletes have ended their careers with one false move in the weight room, so this is an area where it is absolutely critical to get good advice. By good advice we mean from a qualified coach or trainer; books can give you general pointers about fitness, but they cannot replace hands-on advice from a professional who is observing your technique.

- **Cross train.** Cross training, using a sport other than your own, is a great way to stay in top shape. Suppose you're a volleyball player and you also swim or do aqua exercise. In the pool, you get cardiovascular training and you also work all your muscles—without the pounding your body takes on the court. Psychologically, it's refreshing to work out in a different and less competitive environment.
- **Make good use of the off-season.** During the season, you have to think about getting ready for the next competition. But your off-season is an opportunity to step back and look at the big picture. Too many basketball players, for example, just play games during the off-season. But smart players (like Mike) use that time to work on individual skills.

How I Spent My Summer Vacation

Many high school athletes believe that gaining "exposure" to college coaches by participating in Amateur Athletic Union (AAU) and other summer programs is critical to getting an athletic scholarship. But this is not necessarily true.

Marcus Taylor turned his back on AAU basketball in the summer after his junior year. He said he wanted to work on his fundamental skills, prepare for the SATs, and enjoy spending time with his friends. Where did Marcus end up? Being recruited by NCAA champion Michigan State. True, Marcus was way up in the national high school rankings in his junior year. But the point is that he became the number-one recruit in the country on everyone's list by working on his game—not by chasing exposure. Carefully evaluate how you spend summers; use that time to gain the most advantage in your sport and in your life.

Avoid Injury

By making yourself as fit as possible, you reduce your chances of injury and you become more likely to recover quickly if you are injured. But when injuries do occur, how do you deal with them?

It can be OK to play with some pain, such as a lightly sprained ankle; but it's not smart to play with a major injury, such as a broken bone. Sometimes it's hard to tell the difference. Err on the side of caution. Get to know your body and communicate what you're feeling to trainers and doctors. If it doesn't feel right, don't play until you've had an X-ray and have been checked out by a doctor in the appropriate specialty.

Only a few years ago, ACL (anterior cruciate ligament) tears ended careers. Today, medical advances have made it possible to come back even from an injury like an ACL tear. The general principles of fitness apply to rehabilitation as well. Push yourself, but don't overdo it to the point where you risk reinjury. Pay attention to the details.

Win the Mind Game

You can control your thoughts and even your emotions to maximize your performance and get the edge. You can put yourself "in the zone" where you are relaxed but bursting with energy and confidence. You know everything will go right, and it does!

The mind is an amazingly powerful and often untapped resource (and, by the way, the same techniques will help you do well in the classroom and elsewhere). Here are some points to consider before we plunge into how you win the mind game.

- You cannot achieve a goal just by imagining it. Sports psychology works best when you've prepared yourself to excel by taking care of all the other elements we've talked about: nutrition, rest, fitness, and, of course, practicing hard.
- Just like physical skills, psychological skills need to be practiced.
- Every athlete is different; every athlete has his or her own combination of mental skills to maximize performance.

The following sections sketch briefly some of the psychological skills that can lead to athletic success.

Visualization

A surefire way to screw up is to picture the wrong outcome. Keep telling yourself, "Don't hit the golf ball into the water," and the next thing you'll see is a splash. That's because your subconscious mind can't cope with the command "don't." When your parents tell you not to do something, you might immediately see yourself doing that very thing.

Visualize the outcome you want. See the ball falling into the cup, the foul shot dropping through the rim, the tennis ball clearing the net and landing exactly where you want it go. In addition to visualizing a particular act, you can picture a larger situation. For example, imagine yourself playing your best in the biggest game of the year.

Before using visualization (or any of these psychological techniques) in competition, practice them as you would any other skill. For the best results to occur, you need to be relaxed. Athletes often incorporate this kind of mental imagery into their relaxation routines. You can allow yourself to become totally relaxed through a technique such as alternately tensing and relaxing various muscle groups, and then you can visualize playing the game of your life.

Concentration

Have you ever wondered how a basketball player can sink a free throw when everyone in the crowd behind the backboard is waving those long skinny balloons? A superior athlete can "park" his or her mind solely on the task at hand and be undistracted by anything else. Identify the aspects of your sport that require concentration and practice concentrating on them.

It's particularly important not to be distracted by previous difficulties. Tiger Woods's approach to golf demonstrates this point. Tiger has a remarkable ability to recover from the bad shots and bad holes that can ruin a round or an entire tournament for many players. Tiger just focuses on each swing. Like Satchell Paige, he doesn't look back. He looks ahead to whatever can affect his score from that point forward.

Self-Confidence

Do you get nervous before a competition? Are there butterflies in your stomach (or are you throwing them up)? Almost every athlete worries about playing well and fears making mistakes. Some professional athletes who seem completely calm agonize before a game, but they've learned how to harness their nervous tension. Some anxiety or arousal is productive and necessary: if you are completely relaxed, you're asleep!

You can control your tension and go into competition aroused and ready to win. Self-confidence is related to self-talk, a silent conversation you have with yourself. Instead of constantly putting yourself down, think about how prepared you are and see yourself winning. It's the logical outcome of all your preparation.

Sometimes athletes put undue pressure on themselves; they want to win so badly that the prospect of losing literally becomes a nightmare and keeps them awake at night. If you find yourself feeling terrible a lot of the time because of your sport, talk with your parents or your coach. Sports should be challenging but fun. Perspective helps: only one team wins the championship, only one runner wins the race. If you have played your best, you are a winner.

Mental Preparation

What you think is just as important a part of your routine to prepare for competition as getting enough sleep and eating properly. You might find that visualizing success works for you, or that positive self-talk is your secret weapon. Every person is different. Some listen to mellow music to get them ready, others need to hear the music blasting. Try taking a few deep breaths to help you relax right before the game. Some teams have a group cheer or huddle before heading onto the field to help focus their collective tension.

The Big Fix

In striving to get the edge in sports, we've said there is no quick fix. But put together all the elements—practice, conditioning, nutrition, rest, and the mind game—and each adds to the effect of the others. You end up, over a period of time, with the Big Fix.

PART TWO

The High School Years

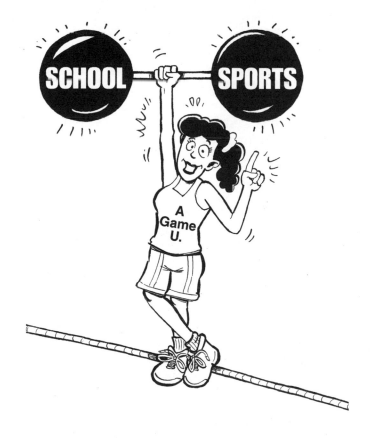

CHAPTER 5

Enjoy High School and Succeed

High school sets the tone for the rest of your life. If you're not happy with the tone you've set so far, there's still time to change direction. The first step is to read this chapter.

The challenge of being a high school student is to learn how to have fun and grow up at the same time. How can you enjoy being a kid while becoming an adult? How can you cope with additional responsibilities in your life?

This chapter will help you step back and gain some insight into your high school years. One of the first things to focus on is the opportunity high school gives you to learn and to develop skills that will enable you to keep learning for the rest of your life.

Learn or Get Burned

As a high school student, you are surrounded by teachers (don't panic!) who spent four years in college, maybe went to graduate school, read umpteen books, did countless hours of research—all to prepare themselves to give you information and insight. You could say, "No, thanks, I'm not interested." Or you could grab all the knowledge you can.

Maybe you don't believe science, math, literature, history, geography, or the ability to speak foreign languages are all that necessary. But think about the value knowledge has in your sport.

Could you be a basketball player without knowing what a pick-and-roll is? Does a baseball player have to know about the squeeze play? Do football players need to know about the draw play, do swimmers need to know about stroke mechanics, do runners need to know about pace? Knowledge plays the same role in the game of life. Without knowledge, you're lost.

Take history, for example. History helps you understand where you are now. It documents the past events that have shaped your community, your society, and even who you are, and it yields clues about the future.

There's No Use Blaming the Teacher

You might think that some of your teachers are not very good at teaching. You might be right. Not all teachers are equally committed to their profession: there are great teachers and there are average teachers. There are teachers who've become burnt out and discouraged, and they've stopped trying. There are some who have a knack for making fascinating material boring beyond belief.

Students who are not doing well in a course often blame the teacher. Even if your teacher is bad, that's a mistake. If you don't learn, the teacher doesn't pay the price: you do. Ultimately, you're responsible for figuring out how to learn the material—whatever it takes.

The Mystery of Homework

Homework might seem like a mystery to you, and you might wonder, "Why do teachers assign homework in the first place?"

Teachers assign homework because . . . (select one)

a) They want to make your life miserable.
b) Reading 30 book reports makes their weekend.
c) They don't realize *South Park* is on TV tonight.
d) It's required punishment for original sin.
e) None of the above.

Is it possible that teachers pile on homework to help you learn and be prepared? Does that mean you should think it's important enough to do—even if it means postponing surfing waves, channels, or the Internet?

You might not like homework, but it plays an important role. Think about the phrase, "Do your homework." It's come to mean, "Be prepared"—whether you are talking sports, business, or school. When someone says, "She does her homework," they are describing a person who is ready to succeed in any area.

Novelist Walker Percy said, "You can get all A's and still flunk life." Those of you who get poor grades may be nodding your heads and saying, "Yeah. I'd rather be street smart than book smart." You might even resent nerds and bookworms who ruin the curve. The reality is most students who get A's are doing just fine. Those with street smarts and good grades do best in life.

The study habits you develop doing homework will come in handy too. There's a huge body of knowledge beyond street smarts or homework. Most of it can be found in books, magazines, and newspapers. If you learn to enjoy reading and make it a habit, you'll learn and be entertained at the same time. But one problem with reading is that it cuts into music, TV, and video-game time. We all need diversions. But how many hours a week do you spend watching TV and playing video games? What do you get out of it? Does it help you achieve your goals?

Choose to Be Smart

Look at our society. You might think it's divided by race, gender, or wealth. There is some truth to that view. But did you ever stop to think that the main division in our society is between People of Smart Persuasion and People of Dumb Persuasion?

You aren't born with a predisposition for one category, but as you grow and mature you gravitate toward one or the other. It's up to you to determine where you belong.

What Does It Take to Join the Smart Persuasion?

It's simple: read. More than anything else, it's exactly what you are doing right now.

If you don't read, you learn only from your own experience. But in a lifetime of reading, you learn from the experience of thousands of other people as well. You can draw upon world-class experts in every field: sports, politics, business, philosophy, religion. Reading about the topics and people that interest you helps you define your goals and develop a plan for accomplishing them. You can read books about Michael Jordan, Tiger Woods, Colin Powell, Oprah Winfrey, Denzel Washington—even George Washington. Once you get drawn into a well-written book, watching a typical TV show seems as pleasant as a visit to the dentist.

Does reading depend on race, gender, or money? No. Reading is for everybody.

Sometimes reading gets a bad reputation, from instances when books are forced on us. People associate reading with being told, "You must study pages 34 to 67 in your dusty old history textbook by tomorrow." Even the vastly talented People of the Smart Persuasion have a hard time reading material that's flat out boring.

Nobody likes being told what to read, even if it's a great book. Your teacher tells you to read the first chapter of *Moby Dick,* and you're already thinking CliffsNotes. It shouldn't have to be that way. Many books are exciting, especially when you're reading them because you want to.

As an athlete, you've got to love a magazine like *Sports Illustrated.* It's one of the best-written publications in the world. Also try opening up your local newspaper or a national newspaper like *USA Today.* You'll find articles and opinion pieces that interest, provoke, and even outrage you. Look beyond the sports section: you'll find fascinating stuff that opens your mind and ensures your place among the People of Smart Persuasion.

When you're out of shape, it's hard to drag yourself to the gym. But when you're in the habit of exercising and you're seeing the benefits, it's hard not to work out. It's the same with reading. Once you get in the habit, you're hooked. You can't stop. You might want to act dumb, but it's hard. You've absorbed so much knowledge, and you can't help thinking about what you read and talking about it with other people. Next thing you know, you're hanging with people who read, who think, who have ideas. You've joined the People of Smart Persuasion.

Be a Computer Jock

Computer literacy is second only to literacy in English for success in our society. It is a requirement for most good jobs. It enables you to efficiently write, analyze, calculate, and file. It gives you access to the

Internet and the ability to benefit from this huge and ever-growing stockpile of information. If you haven't already become proficient at using the operating system, a word program, spreadsheets, and other programs that correspond to your interests, such as graphics or music, now's the time to start.

Touch typing is one of the fundamental skills that give good computer jocks the edge. Touch typists are fast typists, because they use all their fingers and don't have to look at the keyboard. Touch typing is an essential skill for success in college and career. You just won't have the time to hunt and peck. We strongly recommend that you take a typing class. In addition, there are inexpensive self-training computer programs. Many are like video games: you kill the enemy by hitting the right keys. At last—a video game parents can't protest.

Stay Eligible to Play

Playing sports is a privilege, not a right. If you are not doing well academically, most schools and state athletic associations will not let you participate in sports. For example, at many high schools, you have to maintain a grade point average of 2.5 with no grade below a C. If you are getting a D in a course, you may be kicked off the team until you improve your grade.

Clearly, to maintain your eligibility to play, you should know what your school's academic standards are. Then, don't aim for the minimum. If you do, and miss slightly, your playing days are at least temporarily over.

One Sport or More?

How many sports should you play in high school? There are good reasons to play just one; there are also good reasons to play several.

The logic of specializing in one sport is that you can put all your time and energy into getting better in that sport. In the off seasons, you can work on fundamentals and conditioning especially tailored for that sport. Many coaches will tell you that you are more likely to improve and win an athletic scholarship if you play only the sport they are coaching. Another reason you might want to stick to just one sport is to give yourself time to pursue hobbies, extracurricular interests such as music or drama, or a sport not available at your school.

What if you want to play more than one sport because you get fun, satisfaction, and companionship from several? Our general advice is go ahead and do it. One coach, or even your parents, may put pressure on you to play just one sport, but the argument that otherwise you won't do well is not necessarily true. Many of the greatest athletes have been multiple sports athletes. Skills learned in one sport are often transferable to another. And if you can't make decisions in high school based on having fun, when can you?

How to Handle the Pressure

There's pressure to win in sports. The pressure may come from your coach, your teammates, your fellow students, your parents, or yourself. If you like to compete, you'll probably respond well to the pressure. Athletes with a strong desire to win understand that practicing hard and playing hard are absolute necessities. Even if it's difficult or boring at times, they see the value of hard work in the big picture.

Again, the pressure can come from outside, but you'll get the best result when you respond to your own pressure to excel and you block out the outside pressures. Think of a good foul shooter with the game on the line. Opposing fans may be screaming and waving streamers. The shooter hears nothing, and she sees only the rim. Winning in athletics and in life means focusing on the task at hand.

How to Deal with Problems

Satisfaction in athletics carries over to other aspects of your life, and vice versa. You can't really separate them. So if you find yourself troubled by something in athletics or otherwise, ask yourself why. We all have a tendency to put off problems, hoping they will go away. But deep down, you know they won't. So don't let a problem get you down without trying to do something about it. There may not be an immediate solution. But you'll feel better knowing that you've identified the problem and that you're taking steps to solve it.

Keep a Positive Attitude

It's easy to get depressed or angry when things don't go your way. In your sport, you may think the referees made some horrible calls.

Maybe those calls even cost your team the game. But when you step back and look at the situation, can you really say it was a bad call that cost you the game? Or would better execution overall have given you a victory? In sports, bad calls have a tendency to even out. The same goes for life. You may not always get what you want, but if you keep working hard, eventually you'll catch some breaks. The key is not to get bent out of shape when things don't go your way. Keep a positive attitude and keep up the hard work.

Be Open with Your Parents

Your parents (or other advisors) have your best interests at heart. That's why they told you not to eat candy before dinner, or to do your homework before you turn on the TV. If they didn't care about you, they wouldn't bother. Nevertheless, lots of young people ignore their parents' advice. Big mistake. Your parents have lived a lot longer than you have, and they want to give you the benefit of their experience. You may not follow all their advice, but you can only gain by listening to it and considering it.

Do you think your parents are too inflexible in their efforts to get you to do what's right? That's possible. Still, try to be open to your parents' advice and be open with them about your thoughts and feelings. You can learn from each other. Just keep in mind who has the edge in experience. When you are 45 years old, who do you think will have a greater understanding of life: you, or your teenage children?

Go to College

What's the connection between college and success?

- If you want to continue competing in your sport after high school, college is the place to be. It's where you can get the coaching, the competition, and the support from fellow athletes necessary to reach your potential.
- By continuing in your sport, you can further develop habits such as hard work, discipline, cooperation, and confidence that will help you in whatever you do.
- College is where you are trained to deal with information. Most

good jobs require a college degree. For many, flipping burgers is the only alternative to getting a college education.

- At college, the greatest opportunity to learn is outside the classroom. At most campuses you can meet people of varied backgrounds, from all over the country and the world. You can discover a wide range of knowledge that will benefit you for the rest of your life.

CHAPTER 6

Manage Your Time

High school athletes are in a perpetual struggle to balance academics and sports. But life is not simply a balancing act between two pursuits. It's more of a juggling act. You might be juggling school work, sports, responsibilities at home, and maybe a part-time job. As you get older, the juggling act continues. The balls might represent career, family, social, religious, or political obligations, leisure and recreation, and so on. Time management helps you keep all the balls in the air at once.

In high school your time is largely accounted for. Even when you want to goof off after a long day of school and practice, your parents will probably suggest (you might call it *nag*) that you get off the phone, do your homework, clean your room, take the garbage out, and go to sleep at a reasonable hour. In college, you'll be on your own, with far more to do.

No One Is a Natural

Being organized—which involves keeping your goals in mind, staying on top of things, anticipating demands on your time, and planning accordingly—is one of the most important skills you can learn. We say *learn* because no one is born with this ability. Think back to when you were a little kid and your parents pleaded with you to pick up your toys. You probably cried, not realizing the benefit you'd get the next time you wanted to play. If you've already mastered organization, great. If you're like most of us, however, learning to be organized will be either very hard or downright difficult. But once you get into the habit of doing things the right way, you'll never want to return to Disorganization Hell.

Plan for a Lifetime

By combining *life* with *time,* the word *lifetime* reminds us that we're not here forever. There may be an infinite number of things to do in life, but there are a finite number of hours, days, weeks, months, and years in which to do them.

That doesn't mean you have to compulsively schedule every second, or that you can't have any fun. It does mean that, to accomplish your goals, you have to plan your time.

We're sure you remember more than one weekend when you had to write a paper or cram for a test instead of playing sports or going to a movie with friends. Why? Because you hadn't planned to get your schoolwork done. You might have wasted a lot of time watching TV earlier in the week, which was nowhere near as much fun as the activities you had to miss that Saturday when you were home cramming for your test. Even quality goofing off requires planning!

Whole books have been written about time management, but the basic idea is simple: figure out what your priorities are and make sure you put the bulk of your time into those areas. Sometimes you have to handle an unexpected task that wasn't on your priority list, such as when your brother is locked out of the car and you have to bring him the spare set of keys. But if unexpected tasks are always cropping up and you're always reacting to events, you aren't in control of your time.

Think about your last few weeks. Did you spend most of your time "putting out fires" rather than accomplishing your objectives? If so, try to figure out what you can do to change the situation. It will probably help if you talk about the problem with your parents, a coach, a teacher, or a friend.

Start with a Date Book

Do you know what you will be doing next Tuesday at 4 P.M.? Or four weekends from now? The first step in taking control of your time is to get a date book, if you don't already have one.

Date books come in many styles and in a range of prices, including electronic organizers. Get one that works for you and fits your budget. If you tend to lose things, don't invest a lot of money in an electronic organizer. If you use a computer on a daily basis, consider one of the organizer programs that allows you to print out pages from the date book. If you prefer paper date books, go to an office supply store and pick a book that seems best for you.

Some people think they don't need a date book because they're under the illusion they can remember all their tasks and appointments. If you hardly ever do anything, that could be true. If you already have a busy life, a date book will be key to keeping it organized and staying focused on your priorities.

Now, here's the big secret: merely owning a date book does not organize your life any more than owning a textbook prepares you for your final exam. You've got to open your date book, frequently! Keep it with you, even in your gym bag, and use it on a daily basis to record homework assignments, practices, games, work, social appointments: everything you do. You'd be amazed at how easy it is to schedule two activities at the same time if you don't check your date book.

Once you've filled the pages with things to do, look in the book every evening or every morning, whatever time of day works for you, to be sure that you are carrying out your plans. Once a week spend 10 to 15 minutes with your date book. Review how you've been spending your time and look forward to see if your plans are designed to accomplish your goals. If you're not satisfied, figure out what you need to do and when to do it, then enter that information into your date book.

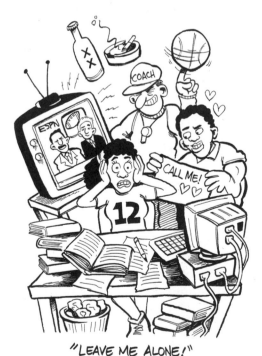

"LEAVE ME ALONE!"

Scrap the Scraps

Imagine that you're out and you don't have your date book with you. You write down an appointment on a napkin, including the address and phone number of where you need to go. You stick the napkin in your pocket, purse, or book bag. Good luck. If all goes well, you remember the appointment and you don't have a conflict. But in the worst-case scenario, you forget all about the napkin and miss the appointment. The next-worst scenario is you remember that appointment, but you don't remember where the napkin with the critical information is. You spend an hour tearing the house apart, then find the napkin in the first place you looked. You have made yourself and your family crazy (and you've possibly uttered a few bad words in your frantic search). Keep your date book with you and use it.

Use a Notebook Too

You have a notebook, or a section of a notebook, for each course you take in school. But how do you record other important information beyond your schoolwork? Here are examples of some of the things you might need to write down.

- You ask your coach to recommend summer workouts that will help you improve your skills, and your coach responds with a series of detailed suggestions.
- Your team is organizing a car wash to raise funds. You're responsible for making the announcements. You've got to write down the date, time, place, price, and other details.
- You're on the phone with a friend who gives you seven possible places to look for a part-time job.
- You go to a presentation on preparing for the SAT. You need to remember dates, places, and the names of some books and some URLs.
- You earn money baby-sitting. You want a record of all the information parents have given you about emergencies, health, food, TV, bed times, and other details that will help you do the best job and make the most money.
- You attend a seminar about selecting a college. You need to keep track of important requirements and deadlines for applications, the Initial-Eligibility Clearinghouse, campus visits, and other information.

None of this data quite fits in your date book. And you already know that scraps of paper are a losing formula. Many successful people keep a separate notebook for this kind of information. They know that they will have to look in only one place to find their notes, no matter what the topic. When the notebook is full, they put it on a bookshelf where they can always go back to it; then they start another one. Each time you start a notebook, put the beginning date on the cover; when it's full, add the ending date.

Keep It Simple

At the beginning of every school year, I would come up with the most detailed system of time management. I'd schedule every minute of my day, take notes on every word my teacher said in every class, come home and recopy my notes, and study four hours every night. I would follow this plan religiously—for about two weeks. Then I'd mess up one day. Suddenly, I'd go from total plan to no plan, like someone on an extreme diet who cannot recover after one lapse.

Make a reasonable plan that you can realistically stick to. Schedule time when you can do anything you want and feel good about it, not guilty. If you see your date book as a tool to help you get the most out of life, you'll want to act on what you've written down.

Getting organized and staying organized is a lifelong effort, but it's an effort well worth making. If you lapse, don't give up any more than you would if you made a bad pass or took a hurdle off the wrong foot. Keep working to improve your organizational skills.

PART THREE

The College Preparation Game

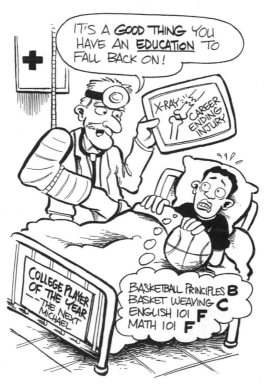

CHAPTER 7

Select the Right College and the Right Coach

If you enjoy school and learning, preparing for college will be relatively easy. You won't have to be concerned about meeting the minimum standards for college entrance: you'll be far above them, and most colleges will be open to you.

Preparing for college is important, so don't let yourself be sidetracked by peers who don't share your goal of getting into a good school. No one comes along and says: "Just be stupid. Don't learn anything, and don't prepare for college." Instead, they throw you curve balls. Maybe they invite you to a party. You say you can't go because you've got a test the next day and you need to study. But they put the pressure on you: "Come on. This party's gonna be cool." They don't even have to say the rest of their message, that studying is not cool. You don't want to be a nerd, you want to be one of the guys. So you let yourself get sidetracked.

This is just one instance, but there will be others as you prepare for college. And sometimes that curve ball has a little extra spin on it: rather than an invitation to a party, it's an invitation to get high or get drunk. How you respond comes back to who you are and who you want to be.

Wherever you go to college, the purpose is to get the best education possible, experience new things, and prepare to go out and succeed in the real world. If you plan to play sports in college, there are many options to choose from—from big-time college basketball on national TV, to lacrosse played in front of friends and family standing on the sidelines, to team sports such as volleyball and hockey, to individual sports such as wrestling and track and field.

Get a Perspective on Recruitment

Being recruited to play sports in college is a status symbol, like having the right sneakers. Friends ask, "Are you being recruited?" You may want to say, "Yeah!" as one of those athletes in demand. Well, we hate to burst your bubble, but recruiters are not fat guys with red suits and white beards carrying bags full of athletic scholarships. Recruiters may care about you as a person, but their job is to sign up athletes who will help their teams win.

From your point of view, selecting the right college is what it's all about, whether you are being recruited or not. You—and not the college recruiters—must decide which college you will attend. Recruiters will show interest only if you can contribute to their athletic programs. But it's up to you to select a college that serves your best interests at the same time. In the hoopla surrounding recruiting, it's easy to lose sight of this fundamental point.

You may be a high school superstar who is actively recruited by big-time colleges. Or you may want to continue your sport in college even though you know you're among the majority of athletes who will never make the cover of *Sports Illustrated*. Perhaps you are already a student in a two-year college and you want to transfer to a four-year school. No matter what your situation, the information in this chapter will help you achieve your goals.

Look, Mom, No Athletics!

Pick a school you would like even if there were no sports. That's what dozens of athletes and coaches told us when we asked them, "What advice about selecting a college would you give to your son or daughter?"

The biggest mistake you could make in selecting a college would be to ignore this advice. Things can change quickly in your sport. The coach could leave. You could be injured. Another athlete could take your spot. You could suddenly find yourself out of competitive athletics, at a college you selected only for its athletic program. You might look around and discover you hate the place. Socially and academically, it's not the college for you. Transferring to another college may not always be the answer. If you transfer, the NCAA may punish you by taking away one or even two years of your eligibility to play your sport. And, the new school may not accept some of your hard-earned credits.

Ask the Right Questions

Which college do you want to attend? The way to find the right school is to ask yourself a lot of questions. We've developed a list that you can use as a starting point to help you figure out which college is best for you and to eliminate schools that don't meet your needs. These questions were suggested by college athletes and coaches, but you should add your own questions to the list. Focus on the questions that will help you get the big picture when it comes to college, and don't get lost in the details.

These questions are in three categories: athletics, academics and career preparation, and social life. Balance all three of these categories to come up with a picture of the right school for you.

Most of these questions are easy to answer. But with some, the answers are not always obvious. Later on, we'll give you some ideas on how to go about it. The first step is to start asking. Here are the questions.

Athletics

- Is the system right for me? Will I fit in with the team's strategy or will I be like a passing quarterback in a running offense?
- Will I be comfortable with the coach's approach to practice?
- Will I be comfortable with the coach's approach to discipline?
- Will I be able to develop my athletic ability as fully as possible in this program?
- How does my ability compare to this school's program? Do I want to be in a big-time program, even if I may not start or star, or do I want to be a top performer on a team at a lower level?
- When recruiting, do representatives of this college one-sidedly praise my athletic ability? Do they make promises about playing time and about not recruiting other athletes at my position? Should I believe such promises?
- Do recruiters say that their program will increase my chances for a pro career? How do I feel about that as a recruiting technique?
- Will I be happy at this college if the coach leaves?
- Is this school under investigation for possible violations of NCAA rules? If so, what are the probable outcomes, and when? How might that affect me?
- How long has the coach been at the school? Under what

circumstances did the coach leave his or her previous job? Was the coach fired or did he or she accept a better job?

- What is the coach's win–loss record? What are this college's expectations about winning? If the team doesn't win, will the coach be fired?
- How much turnover is there among assistant coaches?
- Has the coach ever not renewed an athletic scholarship solely because of poor performance or injury?

Academics and Career Preparation

- What is the right major for me? Does this college have a department in that major that will suit my needs?
- Is the academic level at this college too demanding for me? Will I be in over my head? Or is it not challenging enough?
- Does this school accept athletes who meet the NCAA minimums for eligibility, or are their requirements stiffer?
- Does the coaching staff believe that academics are important or just something that may get in the way of eligibility? What happens if pressure to win conflicts with educational demands?
- Will this college evaluate my academic level? If I need courses to get up to speed, are they available?
- Is tutoring available for athletes? Are there required study periods? If so, is that something I want?
- What is the graduation rate among scholarship athletes in my sport?
- How well prepared are graduates for careers? Does the school keep athletes eligible with easy majors that do not prepare them to compete in the world beyond sports?
- Do former team members have good jobs? Are they advancing in their careers?

Social Life

- Do I want to be in a college located near home? Or do I want to go somewhere farther away? Is there a particular area or climate I'd like?
- Do I want to be in a big city, or on a campus with a beautiful natural setting?
- What is the makeup of the general student body—economically, ethnically, geographically? Will I be comfortable there?
- What about the people on the team? Are they people I'd select as friends?

- How many students attend this college? Would I be more comfortable in a small college, where I might get more individual attention? Or do I want the resources, activities, and diversity that a big college offers? Is there a way to get individual attention even if the college is large?
- Are the students at this college mainly into athletics? Or are they into partying, into studying, into religion? Or does it depend on the group they hang out with?
- How do athletes and the other students get along? Are they isolated from each other or is there lots of interaction?
- How much will it cost to attend this school, beyond my athletic scholarship or whatever other financial aid I receive? What are the indirect expenses, such as transportation and spending money?

Now that you've answered all the questions, you can create a picture of a college that has everything you want. But in real life, there is no such college, for there are no perfect colleges. Each college will have some features you like and some you don't. There's no point in trying to match a college to your every preference. Find a college that you are comfortable with.

Divide What You're Looking for into Three Areas

To select the best college for you, divide what you want into three areas. Figure out what you *must have;* then consider what *would be nice* but would not matter all that much. Between those extremes, place features that are *important* but that you could live without. Make a list of the items in each category. Rule out any college that doesn't have all the items in your must-have section. Then, consider your list of important features. Finally, look at the list of features in your "would-be-nice" category.

Here's an example of this approach, as used by senior basketball sensation Joe Shott. Joe is one of the most highly recruited high school basketball players in the country, and there has been a lot of speculation about which college will win his talents.

When Joe started thinking about where to go to school, TV exposure was the main thing on his mind. He wanted to be on a team with lots of nationally televised games, so millions of people could catch his act. He wanted a team with cool uniforms, so he'd dazzle all his high school buddies. He saw himself going to the NBA after his sophomore season.

In ninth grade, basketball was all Joe could think about. In eleventh grade, Joe blew out his knee. For the first time, playing basketball was not part of his life. While Joe was recovering, his English teacher turned him on to the world beyond basketball. He got excited about reading and writing. The English teacher sponsored a club that produced videotapes. Joe got into that, too; it was fun to do and learn more about.

Over time, Joe saw the problem in holding out for a dream that might or might not come true. He didn't want to be left out in the cold if he couldn't make it as a professional athlete. He saw an athletic scholarship as an opportunity to get a free college education; if everything worked out, he could have a legitimate chance to play in the NBA. Joe decided to prepare himself for a career in communications and work toward becoming a professional basketball player. He developed this picture of an ideal college.

Must Haves
- a good communications major
- a Division I basketball team that likes to run
- a top-20 team with a strong chance to make it to the Final Four
- a head coach who believes in academics and thinks that good students tend to be smart about basketball, too

Importants
- a large university where athletes and nonathletes mix
- a team that recruits nationally and internationally (Joe lived in one neighborhood all his life, and he wants to meet a wide range of people.)
- a chance to start as a freshman

Would Be Nice
- near mountains and seacoast (Joe has always lived in a flat inland area.)
- in or near a big city
- near to where Joe's aunt (who's a great cook) lives
- lots of televised games, cool uniforms

Joe compared South Coast State University (SCSU) to this list. SCSU has all the things on his must-have list. The college is known for its fast-break style of basketball. It's also widely respected for its communications department. SCSU has two of Joe's three important features as well. He probably won't be able to start as a freshman. There is a senior who starts at his position who will almost certainly be picked in the first round of the NBA draft. SCSU's coach expects that Joe would start for the three years after that. As for Joe's would-be-nice list, South Coast, as its name suggests, is near the ocean but not near mountains. There is a big city, where Aunt Susan lives, but it's 90 miles away. There are lots of televised games and an endless supply of Mercury shoes and clothes.

South Coast compared well to his ideal picture, so Joe put the school on his short list of three or four colleges from which to make his final choice. It's good to see that one of Joe's must haves shows that he wants a strong education in communications, which could lead to a career after basketball. Another item shows that he wants a coach who supports that goal. Joe hopes to get into the NBA, but he realizes that he has to prepare himself for an alternative.

Joe's ideal picture didn't include items such as remedial courses or tutoring. That's because Joe applied himself to doing well in school. He expects to apply the same discipline to academics in college, which he knows from his older sister will be harder.

Assess Your Athletic Ability

It's tough to be objective about your own ability. Most people overestimate or underestimate their talent. Your best bet is to ask others, "Based on my ability, am I a candidate for an athletic scholarship?" If they say "yes," ask what types of programs they think would offer you one. Ask people who are knowledgeable about you and your sport, whose judgment you respect, and who have nothing riding on the outcome. Your high school coach and opposing coaches might be those people. Ask enough people so that you won't be overly influenced by one strong, but incorrect, opinion.

Learn how to interpret or "read" what people tell you. If your high school coach says, "I think you'll be the number-one point guard on South Coast State's list," her opinion is that they'll offer you a scholarship. If she says, "Well, there's always a chance that SCSU will recruit you," she's probably trying not to hurt your feelings. But her opinion is they won't.

If you feel you aren't a candidate for an athletic scholarship, don't worry. There are many other types of financial aid available, and there are likely to be many colleges where you can play your sport.

Assess Your Academic Ability

Academic success at any college requires consistent hard work. You can help yourself by selecting a college that will encourage your efforts. For example, if schoolwork remains a struggle for you, an athletic scholarship to a college where most of the students come from the top 10 percent of their high school class might not be in your best interest. If you discourage easily, pick a college where the athletic program supports a structured academic environment. You want a program that insists that you go to study hall, makes it easy to get assistance from tutors, and doesn't wait for you to fail. If you're strong academically, select a school that can challenge you with a strong department in your area of interest.

Create a Short List

Use the assessments of your athletic and academic ability when you put together your list of the five or six colleges you want to seriously consider. You might want to take an approach that has worked well for many athletes: list two colleges where the program is right at your level, two colleges where you think you're reaching, and two that you're certain you can count on.

Be sure the college wants you. All the coaches who were talking to Joe Shott wanted to sign him up, but that's not the case with every athlete. Be sure to ask if a coach is offering you an athletic scholarship. You want to know that at least two of the schools on your short list will give you a scholarship. There is no point in making a list of colleges if none of them wants you.

Research Graduation Rates at Your Short-List Schools

Each year, the NCAA publishes information about graduation rates from athletic programs of all Division I, II, and III colleges. This information is sent to high schools, and Division I and II college recruiters are required to give it to you (or to your parents) when you ask for it. Even if you don't ask for it, they are required to give it to you no later than the day before you are offered admission or financial aid.

Select the Right Coach

You'll be under the supervision of a college coach for four or five years. That coach will probably have more impact on your life than any professor or friend. A coach can make your experience enjoyable, stimulating, rewarding—or miserable. How can you find the right coach?

There is no such thing as a perfect coach. Of course you want a coach who can help you improve your athletic performance. But don't stop there. Select a coach you're comfortable with. If you're having a problem or if things aren't going as you expected, you want to be able to talk to your coach. Find a coach whose values you share, and whose personality fits with yours: someone you respect and someone you enjoy spending time with. You want a coach who cares about you as a person—not just as an athlete.

You might be tempted to go to a college because you like the assistant coach who is recruiting you and you want to continue that relationship. But if that's the case, be careful. In some instances, you may be able to develop a relationship with the assistant coach. But some assistant coaches are salespeople who are constantly on the road recruiting athletes. Find out how much time your recruiter spends with the team.

One Size Does Not Fit All

What qualities in a coach are best for you? Some coaches are strict disciplinarians, while others are more easygoing. Some coaches cultivate close relationships with their athletes, while others keep their distance. There is no one method that will work for every athlete. In fact, some coaches vary their style from player to player in order to get the most out of each team member.

A coach may have to speak sharply to one athlete just to be heard, while another might be crushed by the same approach. Basketball player Grant Hill is now a star for the Orlando Magic. When he arrived at Duke as a freshman, he didn't believe he had the talent to compete at the highest collegiate level. So coach Mike Krzyzewski would say, "Grant, you're doing great, you can play." Coach K even involved Hill's peers in building his morale. Christian Laettner, then a senior who became College Player of the Year, would say, "Grant, you're the most talented player on the team."

An impartial coach doesn't necessarily treat everyone the same way. He or she has the athletes' best interests at heart and figures out how to motivate them. That requires being approachable and listening. John Wooden listened to his athletes even about basketball. When they disagreed with him, he was usually right, based on his greater experience. But once in a while even Coach Wooden learned valuable lessons from his players.

The Intramural Option

As you look at colleges and consider what you want to get out of those years, you might decide that even though you love playing your sport, you want to dedicate most of your time and energy to another passion. Maybe you want to gear your studies so you can carry out original research in a scientific field or you want to prepare to start your own business, compose a symphony, or write a book. You can still enjoy your sport at the intramural level. Many colleges have club sports programs where a group of teams play each other. Practice takes far less time than at the intercollegiate level, and there's no travel to eat up your time and energy. Intramural sports offer a physical workout, competition, friendship, and fun. They are a way you can continue to play your sport in college but shift your main focus to other pursuits.

The Story of Kelly Hughes: A Good Coach Makes All the Difference

Kelly Hughes played volleyball in college. Like many of us she had never been an academic whiz, but she knew that education had to be her number-one priority. So she studied hard. She also wanted to have something that at least resembled a normal college experience, even though she was focused on academics and sports.

Kelly never felt that she was on the same page as her coach. When she tried to have a balanced social life, he questioned her dedication to volleyball. When she chose finance as her major, he was not supportive and implied that an easier major would leave her with more time to concentrate on volleyball.

When Kelly played well, the coach patted her on the back and cheered her on. When her game was off, so was the friendship. The coach projected the attitude that Kelly's social worth was tied to how well she played volleyball.

It seemed to Kelly that the coach was focused on winning to the exclusion of all other considerations. After Kelly had knee surgery in her sophomore year, the team doctor advised a few weeks more rest. Although the doctor explained the risks, he left the decision to Kelly, leaving her vulnerable to pressure. The coach talked about the importance of a big game against a conference rival. He said Kelly's teammates were counting on her and implied that she would be letting them down if she was unwilling to play with a little pain. Kelly did not feel comfortable, but she played. She was back under the knife three weeks later. The doctor said she returned too soon.

Even though they were accomplished volleyball players, many team members suffered from low self-esteem as a result of their treatment by the coach. He constantly made snide comments about their weight: "You're looking a little plump," he'd say to one. Or, "It would be terrible to throw away a great career just because you can't lose ten pounds." The coach's approach to motivating his athletes to lose weight included demeaning nicknames. He called one woman "Chubs." Kelly had a naturally slender build, but she saw her friends resort to drastic dieting under this pressure.

Communicate with Your Coach

Kelly was named to the All-Conference team three of her four years, but she felt miserable and couldn't wait for each season to end. When she got up the courage to talk to her teammates, Kelly found that some of them also had doubts about the coach but were afraid to confront a man who had won four national championships and coached the Olympic team. One athlete said, "Some people say he abuses us, but they just don't understand. When he screams at me I know that he wants what's best for me and the team." Kelly thought about quitting or transferring, but she thought that would mean admitting her life was a failure. Today she looks back and laughs at how she measured her self-worth almost totally by the coach. Although the coach was said to run a model program, nobody kept track of the lives of his athletes after college. A few became pro stars. Many failed to graduate; many who did graduate were unprepared for a career or had physical or emotional problems.

Years later, Kelly talked to her former coach about some of these issues. His reaction was, "You never once approached me with your concerns. You can't expect me to be a mind reader." To Kelly, he had seemed unapproachable, driven to win, with no time for anything other than volleyball.

When Kelly thought back to when she was being recruited, she realized she had allowed herself to slide into her unfortunate situation. When she had tried to ask questions, the coach had acted as though he was admitting her to heaven: she wasn't supposed to ask if her angel wings fit. It's unfortunate that Kelly allowed herself to be intimidated. But it's good that she eventually recognized the problem and worked to overcome it.

Kelly played pro volleyball after graduating, and then worked for a sports apparel company. Being away from volleyball made Kelly realize how much it meant to her. She loved playing and studying the game when it was not turned into a grind. She loved the camaraderie and the competition. Kelly volunteered to coach volleyball at a boys and girls club and discovered she loved to teach. She became an assistant coach at a college whose head coach she respected for his dedication to developing players as all-round people. Several years later, Kelly Hughes became the head coach at South Coast State University.

Pressure to Win

SCSU gave a good sales pitch on the importance of academics, but it was obvious to Coach Hughes that winning was priority number one for the boosters and administrators. When her team finished in the middle of the Conference several years in a row, Coach Hughes was criticized for refusing to offer scholarships to some top high school players even though they met the minimum NCAA standards.

Coach Hughes emphasized academics and moral character as well as athletic talent. She showed her players that they could be students and athletes, and she sold them on the dangers of taking shortcuts. She was highly respected by her former players, who became the program's best salespeople. They spread the word that Coach Hughes was demanding about volleyball and academics because she really cared about her athletes.

Gradually her teams grew stronger and began to attract the best high school players. Not only did she graduate top students, but South Coast became a powerhouse in college volleyball, winning three championships in five years.

Success Breeds Higher Expectations

The boosters started taking championships for granted. They'd get down on Coach Hughes if she did not win, and they even expected undefeated seasons. After three top players graduated, hopes for continued success rested heavily on freshman Jill Pine, who had been one of the all-time great high school stars. Jill had gotten good grades in high school and Coach Hughes had been straightforward with her about the need to be a serious student in college.

When Jill got to South Coast she applied herself—to volleyball and partying. She quickly became one of the top college volleyball players, leading her team to an undefeated season heading into the NCAA

Tournament. On the day before the first tournament game, the coach discovered that Jill had been cutting classes and not turning in assignments. She suspended Jill from the team for the rest of the season, despite protests from boosters, fans, and other players. Number-one ranked South Coast lost in the first round. Coach Hughes explained that under no circumstance would she compromise Jill's education to satisfy those who care only about wins and losses. It was more important to teach Jill Pine the lesson that academics came above all else.

At first Jill was furious and wanted to quit South Coast and transfer to another school where, in her estimation, they were more serious about volleyball. Senior team members convinced her to stay and study. Jill, now a physician practicing sports medicine, credits Coach Hughes for turning her life around.

Get Information on Colleges

There are books that summarize information about all the colleges in the United States. They list where the college is, the type of campus (whether it's city, suburban, or rural), the number of students, the majors offered, tuition and costs, the athletic programs, the extracurricular activities, the types of students who attend, the admission requirements, and other information.

These books may be available in your high school library or in the guidance or college counseling office. Or you can find them in your public library. Things change, so be sure to use a recent edition.

Collegiate Directories publishes a complete listing of collegiate sports programs, coaches, addresses, and phone numbers called *The National Directory of College Athletics.* There are editions for male and female programs. This is a great resource for athletes who want to contact coaches. (You can order a copy by calling 1-800-426-2232 or by visiting their Web site at www.collegiatedirectories.com.)

It's never too soon to start thinking about where you want to go to college. Visualize yourself attending the college of your choice: walking around on campus, going to classes, and competing in your sport. Your vision will motivate you to work hard to get there.

Pick a School You Would Like Even If There Were No Sports

You say we've said this already? OK! You remembered the main principle of selecting the right college for you.

CHAPTER 8

The Financial Aid–Scholarship Game

If you're offered an athletic scholarship, should you accept it? "What?" you may ask, "Why not? An athletic scholarship is the ideal. It pays for my whole college education and when I'm finished with school I won't have student loans to pay back. How can you beat that?"

Maybe you can't. An athletic scholarship (technically called a *grant-in-aid*) has many advantages and may be the best way for you to finance college. But it also has its disadvantages. For example, did you know that athletic scholarships are renewed one year at a time and are not always renewed? Today's ideal can become tomorrow's disaster. In this chapter, we'll talk about the advantages and disadvantages of scholarships in detail.

Here's another generally unknown fact about athletic scholarships: they don't pay for your whole college education. Partial athletic scholarships are more common than full athletic scholarships, or what are known as *full rides*. Partial scholarships are often given in percentage terms, such as 40 or 60 percent of a full ride, or in fractional terms, such as a one-quarter or one-third scholarship. Even full athletic scholarships fall short of paying for the entire cost of attending college, because they don't cover incidental expenses and other costs that can amount to several thousand dollars a year.

Our advice is that you don't focus solely on athletic scholarships: instead, research and consider *all* forms of financial aid. That way, you'll be able to make an informed decision based on all your options.

The Goal

College is a great investment, but it can be an expensive one. It costs over $120,000 to attend many highly competitive private colleges for four years. Our society needs and values education, so there are many financial aid programs sponsored by governments, foundations, service organizations, professional associations, companies, unions, and religious institutions. An athletic scholarship and/or other kinds of financial aid can go a long way toward paying for your college education.

Mom! Dad! Help!

Determining the best financial aid package for you—and how to get it—can be difficult and complex. We got a headache trying to translate the rules governing financial aid, and especially the Byzantine language of the NCAA, into plain English. We're not alone. Judges have been to college and law school. They know how to read complex documents. Here's what one judge said about the *NCAA Guide for the College-Bound Student-Athlete:* "It seems to me there's a lot wrong with this. I can understand why they [an athlete and his parents] may have made a mistake, if in fact they made a mistake. Because if you try to read this, you can't interpret what you're reading."

Our goal in this chapter is to give you the information you need to get started on your quest for financial aid. Parents have been dealing with financial information and decisions for at least twice as long as teenagers. And they are probably the ones that will be paying. Seek their help!

What Is an Athletic Scholarship?

NCAA Division I and II colleges are permitted to award athletic scholarships, which are defined as financial aid to athletes who meet the organization's eligibility requirements, regardless of their financial need. Unlike some other forms of financial aid, these are grants, not loans. You don't pay them back. This is a big plus. Just ask a recent college graduate who is faced with a mountain of debt.

Athletic scholarships are awarded one year at a time, and, according to NCAA regulations, "may be renewed each year for a maximum of five years within a six-year period."

Full Athletic Scholarships

One ideal scenario is to get a full athletic scholarship. Here is what the NCAA permits a full ride to cover

- tuition
- fees
- room and board
- required textbooks

The amount awarded for room and board varies. If you live on campus, it depends on factors such as the size of your room, the number of roommates, and your meal plan. If you live off campus, your room and board allowance can be no higher than the average of these on-campus costs at your college.

You'll have expenses beyond the above-mentioned categories (see page 66 for a list of college costs), and a full ride does not cover all the expenses of attending college. Other sources of financial aid, such as the Federal Pell Grant Program, are described later in this chapter.

Partial Athletic Scholarships

The NCAA limits the number of athletic scholarships a college can offer in each sport. For example: Division I-A football can award 85 scholarships; Division I women's basketball, 15; Division I men's swimming 9.9; and Division II women's field hockey, 6.3 (for the number that can be awarded in your sport, see the charts on pages 108–111).

A coach can divide a scholarship to attract more athletes to a team. A typical men's swimming team has 25 swimmers and divers. If the coach uses his 9.9 scholarships to give out nine full rides and one 90 percent scholarship, that leaves 15 slots to fill with no grants-in-aid to offer. The coach is more likely to give out between one and three full scholarships to attract star swimmers, and then divide the remaining scholarships into halves, thirds, quarters, and even smaller segments to fill the three lanes in each event.

Look beyond Division I Schools

High school athletes often have their hearts set on an NCAA Division I school, even if it means not getting much playing time. That may be the right move for you. But you'll never know unless you consider the other options.

Take for example NCAA Division III, which includes top-level academic institutions with excellent sports programs. Devean George, who was picked in the first round of the NBA draft by the L.A. Lakers, played for Division III Augsburg College in Minnesota. Like any college, Division III schools consider athletic achievement as part of the qualifications for admission, but they are not permitted to offer athletic scholarships.

Special Assistance Fund

The NCAA divides $15 million per year among its Division I member colleges to pay the expenses of student athletes beyond what is covered by athletic scholarships. To be eligible, an athlete must either have received a Pell Grant or demonstrate financial need. An athlete can receive up to $500 by submitting receipts. The fund covers expenses such as clothing, emergency travel, expendable school supplies, and medical and dental payments not covered by insurance. Once the funds are received from the NCAA, disbursing them is entirely at the discretion of the college.

The Special Assistance Fund comes from the $216 million per year paid by CBS to televise the men's basketball tournament. In 2003, CBS begins paying $545 million a year for these rights. At that point, the NCAA intends to increase the Special Assistance Fund to $25 million a year, and to increase it 8 percent annually from there. The $500 amount that can be paid annually per athlete will also increase.

Funding Sources Other than Athletic Scholarships

You can go to college with or without an athletic scholarship. The federal government, many states, and colleges themselves offer aid based on financial need. These packages include outright grants, work-study (aid in return for doing a part-time job at the college), and loans.

You need to work hard to find what's available to you. There are billions of dollars out there for people who want to attend college. But because a lot of other deserving students are looking for loans and grants, it's important to start early. Many programs require you to fill out forms that ask for a ton of financial information, and they have strict deadlines (so don't be a day late sending in your application).

- **Pell Grants.** The Federal Pell Grant Program paid college students up to a maximum of $3,125 in the 1999–2000 academic year, depending on financial need. These grants are a boon to any college student short on funds. For recipients of full or partial athletic scholarships, Pell Grants have a special attraction. Unlike most other forms of financial aid, they are not offset against athletic scholarships. That means the college does not subtract the Pell Grant from your grant-in-aid. A Pell Grant can go a long way toward paying for the costs not covered by even a full athletic scholarship. To apply for a Pell Grant, you file a FAFSA, or Free Application for Federal Student Aid (see below).

- **State aid.** All states provide financial aid to college students based on need, and many states also offer awards based on academic achievement (see appendix 3). Many states require a FAFSA; some also require additional financial information on their own forms. The aid is often geared toward students who attend colleges within that state.
- **Organizations.** Get your parents involved: they may belong to unions, churches, or other organizations that offer scholarships.
- **Other aid.** The College Board Web site (collegeboard.org) has a database of thousands of organizations that award financial aid. You enter information about yourself into the search engine, and it pulls up scholarships you may qualify for. There are also printed guides, but the Internet is a far more efficient way to go.

FAFSA: One-Stop Shopping for Federal Aid

How do you first apply for a Pell Grant or any other form of federal aid, such as Stafford loans? By March of your senior year in high school you submit a Free Application for Federal Student Aid (FAFSA). To find out more about federal student aid, the best place to start is the U.S. Department of Education Web site (www.ed.gov/finaid.html). That site puts you one click away from submitting a FAFSA electronically. You can also call toll free at 800-4-FED-AID (800-433-3243).

To renew your federal aid once you're in college, you are required to submit a FAFSA each year. There have been scandals involving athletic departments that "helped" athletes by falsifying documents so their athletes would receive aid for which they did not qualify. Beware! It's your signature on your application, be it electronic or ink, and submitting false information is a federal crime.

Research Your Options

Here is some information that will prove helpful to you as you research your options for college funding.

Learn the Alphabet

To understand your options, you need to know about the organizations that govern college sports. Here is a list. You will also find contact information for these groups in appendix 3. These groups are almost always referred to by their initials.

- National Collegiate Athletic Association (NCAA)
- National Association of Intercollegiate Athletics (NAIA)
- National Christian College Athletic Association (NCCAA)
- National Small College Athletic Association (NSCAA)
- National Junior College Athletic Association (NJCAA)

The NCAA is by far the largest governing body in college sports. A total of 340,000 athletes at 1,040 schools participate in its programs. The NCAA's rules on athletic scholarships and eligibility are the most complex, and there are different requirements for each of its three divisions. Even if you end up attending a non-NCAA school, you'll probably consider the NCAA during your decision-making process. Or you might end up transferring into an NCAA program (see chapter 9 for more on NCAA rules).

College Costs

Here is a checklist of the cost categories you may incur as a student. Not every category applies to every student, but this section can help you budget.

- Tuition (what you pay to attend classes)
- Fees (student government activities fee, laboratory equipment fee, sometimes lumped in with tuition)
- Room and board (what you pay for a place to sleep and food to eat)
- Computer (when you need your own)
- Books and supplies (textbooks, computer supplies, pens, pencils, organizers, date books)
- Transportation to and from school
- Incidentals (laundry, snacks, clothes, entertainment, phone, room decoration)
- Car (gas, insurance, parking, maintenance)

Search Online

The Internet has revolutionized the process of information gathering and it is a strong resource for collecting material on college admissions and financial aid. Web sites with vast amounts of pertinent information include: the College Board Web site (www.collegeboard.org), the U.S. Department of Education site (www.ed.gov/finaid.html), and FinAid (www.finaid.com).

Earning an Athletic Scholarship

Let's say you've decided to go to college, and you think that earning an athletic scholarship is the best way for you to get there. You might believe that to get an athletic scholarship you should concentrate on your sport and meet the minimum academic requirements for college admission. We sincerely hope you reject that strategy because it would deprive you of knowledge. Aside from that, the strategy is only half right.

You do need to work hard to improve your athletic skills rather than rely on raw talent. But you also need to do well in school. Almost every coach says that grades are a critical factor in selecting athletes for scholarships. Coaches refer to athletes who are achieving only the

---

How Is Need Defined?

We mention financial need several times in this chapter. Another term you will hear is *need-based aid*. In this context, exactly what is the definition of *need*?

Need is the difference between two numbers. The first number is the cost to attend your college; the second number is what your family is expected to contribute toward that cost (called the Expected Family Contribution, or EFC). The second number is arrived at by using a formula that includes variables such as family income, family size, and number of other children in college. When you fill out the FAFSA, you and your family need to enter pages and pages of detailed financial information. Don't be discouraged; just take it one step at a time. A college education is worth it.

---

minimum as *academically marginal*. They know that these students are the most likely to flunk out of college or be unable to maintain eligibility. Coaches are afraid to risk scholarships on academically marginal athletes—plus, they wonder if an athlete who won't study the math book will study the playbook or the techniques of his sport.

Evaluate Scholarship Offers: Truth in Aid

A college offers you an athletic scholarship by sending you an award letter. The letter may state that you are being offered a full athletic scholarship, or it may state that you are being offered a partial scholarship and indicate the amount.

You may receive such letters from several colleges. That's a good thing, but it also leads to a problem. Award letters are not uniform. They vary from college to college. Generally, they tell you what you are going to get, but not what you are going to have to pay. That makes comparisons difficult.

Which Is Larger: One Half or One Fifth?

Chris Cardinal wants to play baseball at the collegiate level. Two Division I baseball powers have offered him scholarships. South Coast State University offered Chris a one-fifth scholarship, while Cadwallader College offered him a half scholarship. If Chris must choose solely for financial reasons, which school should he pick? Think about it before reading the next paragraph.

Did you decide you didn't have enough information to answer the question? You're right. Tuition, fees, and room and board at Cadwallader, a private school, come to $30,000 a year. The same costs at South Coast for out-of-state students such as Chris, who have to pay tuition, add up to $16,000. Let's do the math. Half of $30,000 is $15,000. That's what Chris's financial obligation would be at Cadwallader. Four fifths of $16,000 is $12,800. That's what Chris would have to pay at South Coast. In this case, one fifth is better than one half.

The difference is even larger than it appears, because the "incidental" expenses at Cadwallader are higher than they are at South Coast. For one thing, air fare from Chris's home to Cadwallader is about double what is costs to fly to South Coast.

Chris must consider at least one more factor. Some of the nonathletic financial aid he's applying for is partly based on the cost of attending the college in question.

Dare to Compare

You too must go through these calculations to get to the bottom line and find out which college is offering the best financial deal from the point of view of what you and your family will have to pay. This dollars-to-dollars comparison may not be the decisive factor in your decision, but it is certainly an important factor.

To make it easier to find the bottom line, we've created a financial-aid calculator and posted it on A-Game.com. Or you can go through the math by hand. Use a worksheet like the one on the next page for each college you are considering.

After you have gone through these calculations, look at the figure you arrived at for your college cost (item III) for each college. That gives you an apples-to-apples comparison between the actual cost of attendance at the colleges you are considering.

If you need to take out loans, also compare the figures you arrived at for what you will pay (item V). Loans eventually must be repaid. Therefore your college cost line is the most meaningful financial comparison. Of course, if your college cost is more than you can afford, the "what you will pay" line may become the decisive factor.

Don't Be Afraid to Negotiate

You receive a computer-generated award letter, perhaps with NCAA bylaws printed in tiny type on the reverse side, and it creates a certain impression: This is official and final. You ask yourself, "Should I sign on the dotted line?" This is not just a figure of speech, for there actually is a dotted line, or at least a line, for your acceptance signature. But hold on. There is a question to consider before you get to yes or no.

The question is, should you ask for more? Don't shy away from negotiating with the coach. If the coach says no, you can still say yes. But if you decide to negotiate, be graceful about it. Clearly explain why you need more. Your goal is to get a better offer, not to tick the coach off.

For example, let's say a coach offers you an athletic scholarship that's less than a full ride. You have to either accept it or reject it, right? Wrong. You can negotiate for more—especially if they want you badly enough and you have a better offer from another college.

Here's one example of how you might start a negotiation. Remember Chris Cardinal? South Coast offered him a one-fifth scholarship and Cadwallader offered him one half. But, the cost of attending Cadwallader (without incidentals) came to $16,000 and the cost of attending

Financial-Aid Worksheet

Name of College _____

I. Costs

1. Tuition _____
2. Fees (if separate) _____
3. Room and board _____
4. Books and supplies _____
5. Transportation to and from school _____
6. Health insurance _____
7. Incidentals (laundry, snacks, clothes, entertainment, phone, room decoration—or add your own categories) _____
8. Car (gas, insurance, parking, maintenance) _____

Sum = total cost of attendance _____

II. Aid

1. Value of athletic scholarship (grant-in-aid) _____
2. Probable payments from Special Assistance Fund (NCAA Div. I only) _____
3. Federal Pell Grant _____
4. State aid _____
5. Financial aid from college _____
6. Special award #1 _____
   Special award #2 _____
   Special award #3 _____
7. Probable earnings from work-study _____

Sum = total aid _____

III. Your college cost (subtract total aid from total cost) _____

IV. Loans

1. Student loans (Stafford, Perkins, PLUS, etc.) _____
2. Other loans _____

Sum = total loans _____

V. What you will pay (subtract total loans from your college cost) _____

South Coast came to $12,800. Cadwallader is Chris's first choice. But $3,200 makes a difference to Chris and his family.

Chris's father called Mo Jennings, the baseball coach at Cadwallader, and explained the situation. Chris really wants to go to Cadwallader, but unless Cadwallader can come up with another $3,200 he won't be able to.

Chris and his family discovered something by asking Coach Jennings to increase his offer. They discovered they had leverage. The coach needed a left-hander to fill a hole in his pitching staff. He had hoped to get Chris for a half scholarship, but he was prepared to give more. In fact, he offered a 60 percent scholarship. Giving this extra 10 percent didn't mean all that much to Coach Jennings, but every tenth at Cadwallader is $3,000—an amount that meant a lot to the Jennings family. They took the offer, and they might even have gotten the remaining $200 if they'd held out a little longer. They'll never know.

A coach offers you an athletic scholarship for one reason: he or she wants you on the team. Therefore, like Chris, you have leverage. If there is more funding available, you may get it. But only if you ask. Of course, you're in a stronger position to ask if you have another offer in hand that you could happily accept.

How to Maintain Your Scholarship

You have been offered an athletic scholarship at the school of your choice, and you have decided that this is your best route for college funding. But that is not the end of the process. You need to know the story of how scholarships are renewed and how you can safeguard your scholarship.

Athletic Scholarships Are Awarded One Year at a Time

We often get e-mails and phone calls from disenchanted athletes and parents. They thought an athletic scholarship was forever, like love—only to find out that there is no such thing as a guaranteed four-year full ride.

No matter what a coach may imply, NCAA regulations prohibit a college from promising to automatically renew an athletic scholarship. An award cannot be taken away during the school year based on poor athletic performance. A coach can, however, choose not to renew a scholarship. An athlete must be notified of nonrenewal in writing by

The Effect of Need-Based Aid on an Athletic Scholarship

This complex subject applies only to NCAA Division I and II equivalency sports. If you know you will not be in this category, skip this headache.

If you're still here, stay with us—or it could cost you big bucks. The first thing you need to know is the difference between a headcount and an equivalency sport.

Headcount sports exist only in Division I. In a headcount sport, any athletic scholarship, even a small partial scholarship, counts against the maximum number of scholarships permitted by the NCAA. Examples of headcount sports are Division I football and men's and women's basketball.

In *equivalency sports,* fractional athletic scholarships count against the maximum number, but they can be apportioned by the coach. For example, a Division I men's swimming coach could spread 9.9 scholarships, the maximum number allowed, among all 25 swimmers on his team. The tables on pages 108–111 identify Division I headcount and equivalency sports. All NCAA Division II sports are equivalency sports.

Here's the problem. In equivalency sports, need-based financial aid counts against the NCAA maximum number of scholarships when you have athletic aid as well as need-based aid. For example, the coach awards you a half athletic scholarship that comes to $5,000. You are also granted $5,000 in need-based financial aid. You count against the coach's allowable maximum as one full athletic scholarship.

Why might this be your problem? Say the swimming coach discovers after you arrive at college that you will receive the $5,000 in need-based financial aid. He has already awarded all 9.9 athletic scholarships. But your need-based financial aid means he has a half scholarship less to give. He asks you to give up your athletic scholarship for the benefit of the team.

How can you avoid getting such a nasty surprise? First, if need-based financial aid is important to you, you should probably not sign early because you don't yet know how much need-based aid you will receive. Second, don't assume that a coach knows you are applying for or have been granted need-based aid. Tell the coach about your need-based aid and ask if it will have an impact on your athletic scholarship. Then you can factor in this critical information when deciding what college to attend. The same concept applies when you are renewing your athletic scholarship.

July 1, which is a disastrous time to try to get into another college or create another financial aid package.

Many of the questions we receive involve a coach who has quit or been fired. Promises are out the door when a new coach takes over. He has no allegiance to the athletes on the team. He did not recruit them, and they may have contributed to the demise of his predecessor.

If you feel your scholarship may be in jeopardy, ask the coach about your future immediately (well, maybe not right after you drop a pass).

By NCAA rules, an athlete can appeal a nonrenewal to a committee outside the athletic department. There are no NCAA guidelines for these committees, however, so they vary from school to school. At colleges with high ethics and big budgets, committees tend to support athletes if they feel nonrenewal is related only to performance or injury. But they generally support a coach who can show that the athlete violated a team rule or the school's conduct code.

So what happens if an athlete is injured, doesn't make an effort, or fails to live up to expectations for some other reason? Some athletic departments and coaches are more concerned than others about their obligations to athletes. But all coaches are under pressure to win with a limited number of scholarships. Scholarships taken up by unproductive players don't produce victories.

At South Coast, the football coach helps players who are not contributing transfer to colleges that can use their abilities. But last year, he had a sticky situation: a player who was happy at the school and did not want to transfer. The coach started looking for reasons not to renew that player's athletic scholarship that would be acceptable to the appeal committee, such as an academic problem or a violation of college regulations. There have been instances at South Coast where football stars have had their scholarships renewed when they've hardly been to a class or when they were under indictment for a crime. But for an athlete who is not helping the team, flunking one course or breaking a minor dormitory rule might be used as the basis for not renewing a scholarship.

Renewing Partial Athletic Scholarships

Partial scholarships can be abused because they have the potential to be increased. Say you're offered a one-quarter scholarship, and the coach holds out the possibility of a full ride after a couple of other players graduate. This is a slippery slope. Scholarships are not supposed to be pay better for play better. But if you don't perform on the athletic field, the coach might not increase the scholarship.

Safeguarding an Athletic Scholarship

The NCAA denies that having an athletic scholarship is similar to being an employee of the school. But the bottom line is that you are under pressure to perform to earn the financial aid, just as an employee must perform to earn a salary.

Ideally, you'd like to concentrate on your sport and enjoy it without the pressure or distraction of knowing that your ability to stay in college is tied to your performance. How can you safeguard your athletic scholarship? Here are some suggestions.

When You're Being Recruited

- Select a program where the level of competition is realistic for you. If you are a high school superstar and you are big enough and strong enough, that program could be a top Division I team. If you are not a superstar, think twice before joining a program where you are likely to be one of the most expendable athletes.
- Ask recruiters if the program will recommend that your financial aid be renewed each year even if you are injured. The NCAA does not permit recruiters to say that financial aid is automatically renewed. But they are permitted to say that they will always request renewal, and that the financial aid department has always followed their recommendations in the past.
- Ask a coach's current and former players what happens to recruits who don't measure up to expectations. Does the coach renew their scholarships or look for reasons not to renew? Does the coach help them transfer or make their lives miserable so they will quit and free up a scholarship?

When You're in College

- Do your schoolwork and follow the college rules. This is your game plan for success. If you depart from this game plan, you will fall behind and have to play catch-up.
- Practice hard and have a good attitude. Other things being equal, a coach will try to get rid of a "high-maintenance" athlete.
- Protect yourself from illness and injury by taking conditioning seriously and maintaining healthy eating and sleeping habits.

Financial aid and scholarships are a big issue in your college plans. But if you have the will to get an education, you will never be shut out. You need to do your part in searching for funds. Visit your school's college counselor. Get on the Internet. Go to the library. Don't wait for your athletic scholarship to come through: you don't want to be left without the option of attending college because you didn't plan.

No matter how economically deprived you may be, college is an option. You may have to join the Armed Services for a couple of years, work full-time or part-time, fight, scratch, and claw. Yes, it would be easier to have a full ride. But you'll gain a stronger appreciation for your college education if you are the one who makes it happen by your own diligence in securing funding.

CHAPTER 9

Prepare for College: The Details

Now that you have defined what kind of college you'd like to attend, you need to create a solid plan to get you there. Organizing the necessary details is an important part of that effort. This chapter will tell you what you need to know. Addresses and telephone numbers of organizations you may need to contact are included in this chapter (additional resources are in appendix 3).

Know the Rules

The National Collegiate Athletic Association (NCAA) rules most of the kingdom of college sports. It determines an athlete's eligibility to practice and play in college and administers the rules that govern athletic scholarships. You may think that some of the NCAA's rules are unfair or absurd. But like it or not, they are the rules you must live by if you want to participate in NCAA-sanctioned sports. If you don't learn the rules, you could inadvertently break them and place yourself in jeopardy of losing your eligibility or your scholarship.

The first step is to get a copy of the NCAA's free guide. Each year the Association publishes the *NCAA Guide for the College-Bound Student-Athlete*. The rules in effect during your senior year will determine your college eligibility. But there are lots of things in the pamphlet you should know when you're in ninth grade (for example, which high school courses are required for eligibility) so start reading early.

The pamphlet may be available from your high school. If not, you can obtain a copy from the NCAA online, or by phone or mail. You can also use the NCAA Hotline to hear answers to frequently asked questions and to order the *NCAA Guide for the Two-Year Student-Athlete*. (See appendix 3 for contact and ordering information.)

Find the Right Advisors

It's your responsibility to alert your guidance counselor of your intention to play college sports. That way, your counselor can help make sure you take the right courses and prepare properly for college entrance exams.

An advisor might be an expert on college academic requirements, but he or she might not know the intricacies of the NCAA rules. To participate in NCAA-sanctioned athletics as a college freshman, an athlete has to satisfy the requirements of a particular college as well as the requirements of the NCAA. We cannot put enough stress on the importance of understanding exactly what is required of you: find the relevant parts of the NCAA pamphlet, show them to your advisor, and ask questions to make sure you are doing everything necessary to satisfy the NCAA.

Guidance counselors are not the only people who can advise you. Your coach may be able to help. Or talk to a teacher you respect. The teacher will usually be pleased to help.

Compare what one person tells you with what another tells you, and evaluate everything you are told. Even excellent counseling cannot substitute for your own thinking. Spend a lot of time considering all your options and avoid hasty decisions. It's your future, and you are in charge of making it right.

Beyond finding the right advisors, timing is also important. Don't settle for college counseling that doesn't start until junior or senior year. To be sure you're doing everything necessary to be eligible in college, start thinking about these issues when you are in ninth grade.

Take the Right Courses

If you don't take enough *core courses* in high school, you won't be eligible to compete in college. You'll find information about core courses in the *NCAA Guide for the College-Bound Student-Athlete* and from your high school guidance counselor.

Core courses must be academic courses, such as English and math; but not every academic course is automatically a core course. Non-academic courses—such as driver's education, physical education, metal shop, cooking, and sex education—are not core courses. Remedial courses, even if they are in academic areas, are not core courses.

In the NCAA's 1999–2000 guide, the following are the subjects on which core courses must be based: English, mathematics, natural or physical science, social science, and what they term additional academic courses in foreign languages, computer science, philosophy, or nondoctrinal religion. The *NCAA Guide* also tells you how many years of each subject you need.

As an example, to be eligible to participate in athletics at a Division I or Division II college in 1999–2000, you have to successfully complete at least 13 core courses in high school. Your grade point average in those 13 courses must be no lower than 2.0 (a C average). But it pays to get a better grade (aside from the benefit that you'll learn more). As your grade point average moves up, your minimum required college-entrance-exam score for Division I eligibility goes down. Once you get your grade point average to 2.5 (a C+ average), you've reached the maximum benefit in lowering the minimum SAT or ACT scores. Of course, you increase your chances of being admitted to the college and athletic program of your choice by having an average in the 3.0 to 4.0 range (a B to A average).

Take your core courses early and often and don't limit yourself to the minimum number of core courses. Studies have shown that academic success in college has little relationship to SAT or ACT scores, but it is closely related to doing well in lots of core courses. Aim for taking 16 to 20 of them.

The Road to Eligibility

The NCAA has created the Initial-Eligibility Clearinghouse. Behind this catchy title lurks something important to you. To be eligible to participate in Division I or Division II athletics as a college freshman, you must register with the clearinghouse after your junior year in high school.

Use the Student Release Form in the *NCAA Guide for the College-Bound Student-Athlete.* The clearinghouse must certify that you have satisfied grade point average and core-course requirements and achieved the required score on the SAT or ACT. You can then check to see if the clearinghouse has your record on file by telephoning and using the PIN on your Student Release Form.

It is the responsibility of your high school principal to determine which courses qualify as core curriculum courses. Your high school must submit a list of certified core courses to the clearinghouse. If your school does not send athletes into Division I and II programs often, it may not have done this. So if you intend to play in Division I or II, make sure your school has submitted a list of courses. You can go online to find out if your school has submitted courses and to learn what courses are on that list (go to www.act.org/ncaa/). You can get a free copy of the Initial-Eligibility Clearinghouse brochure and form by calling the NCAA Hotline at 1-800-638-3731.

Core Knowledge When You Need It

The clearinghouse hasn't always been adept at handling its responsibility. In one unfortunate case, an athlete who had a 3.5 grade point average and satisfied the SAT requirement packed her bags to leave for freshman orientation. But there was a hitch.

The clearinghouse had not made the final determination. When they finally got around to reviewing this athlete's transcript, they determined that one of her English course did not qualify. This left the unfortunate athlete with 12.5 core courses, 0.5 below the required 13. A legal mess ensued, and the athlete wasted a year battling through this nightmare. Although she finally won the case, it was a hollow victory because the court did not rule until well into the school year.

Clearly, the time to find out what courses will be accepted as core courses is not when you submit your application to the clearinghouse. When you enter high school find out which courses are core courses and plan when you are going to take them. Passing 13 core courses is not difficult if you plan accordingly. Again, this is a minimum standard. You're going to be better prepared for college level work if you've taken 16 to 20 core courses. We feel bad for the girl whose eligibility was overturned, but her problem would not have arisen if she had done more than the absolute minimum.

Partial Qualifier Purgatory

Division I and II athletes who come close to meeting the grade point and the SAT or ACT scores may be eligible to practice but not compete during their freshman year. See the *NCAA Guide for the College-Bound Student-Athlete* for complete details. It is much easier to invest your time in getting good grades and scores than trying to grasp the intricate requirements of partial qualifier status.

Initial Eligibility, Step by Step

These are the basic steps in the process of securing your eligibility.

1. Read "Making Sure You are Eligible to Participate in College Sports," found in the *NCAA Guide for the College-Bound Student-*

Athlete. Ask your college counselors for the Initial-Eligibility registration materials from the clearinghouse. Counselors can call to request materials (319-337-1492).

2. You normally register with the clearinghouse after your final junior year grades are posted on your transcript. High school counselors can waive the $25 clearinghouse fee if you have received a waiver of the SAT or ACT fee.

3. It is your responsibility to make sure the clearinghouse has all the documents it needs to certify you. These include

   - your completed and signed student release form (normally submitted early in your senior year)
   - the fee, unless waived
   - your official transcript, mailed directly from every high school you've attended
   - your ACT or SAT scores

If you're a foreign student, there is a special application with other requirements.

Aim for Good Grades

In the first class of the semester, a teacher asked her students, "What grade do you want?" Just about everyone answered, "an A." Then she asked, "What grade do you plan to get?" There was a big silence. Most students wanted an A, but they were not planning to earn it. Finally, a few students said A, some said B, some said C. You can bet that very few students who planned to get C's ended up with A's.

Your goal should be knowledge, not grades. But there is a relationship between the two. Both require work. You can't just want to get a good grade: you have to plan to get it.

Studying has to be as routine as practicing for your sport is. Study at a regular time and place and avoid distractions. Background music is OK, but you cannot study while talking to a friend on the phone. Many students pretend they are studying while they are actually watching TV. If you believe TV helps you learn, why not apply your theory to sports? Suggest to your coach that your favorite programs be projected on a giant screen during practice.

Perhaps you're having a problem in a class, and you hope that it will go away if you ignore it. It won't. You will just fall further behind.

Ask your teacher for help. If a quick explanation won't solve the problem, the teacher might recommend a tutor.

Success does not necessarily mean getting an A. You may have a terrible time with a particular subject, or you may be digging yourself out of an academic hole. If you honestly give it your best effort and you earn a C, that's success. Savvy coaches and business leaders responsible for selecting personnel seek people who are improving. They know that someone who works hard often overtakes the person who's doing well but running on cruise control. In fact, students who do well without a lot of effort—both in sports or academics—sometimes believe they can get by without hard work. Later on, when the competition gets tougher, they find out they're wrong.

SAT and ACT

When colleges select students, they are increasingly giving more weight to high school records and less weight to scores on standardized tests. The NCAA, however, requires that you take the SAT or the ACT tests to be eligible to participate in NCAA-sanctioned sports in Divisions I and II.

The *NCAA Guide for the College-Bound Student-Athlete* has information about the minimum SAT and ACT scores required for college athletic eligibility. One interesting NCAA rule: you can combine your highest scores on each part of the test, even if they were earned on different test dates. High schools make announcements about when and where the tests are given, or you can check the SAT and ACT Web sites (see appendix 3). You can register online to take the tests.

You can take the SAT or ACT more than once. It's a good idea to take the test for the first time during your junior year. That way, you become familiar with it and you have plenty of time to improve if necessary. Sometimes students put off taking the test because they can't afford the fee. Fee waivers may be available for students from families with low incomes. Ask your counselor.

How can you improve your SAT or ACT scores? Your high school may have a program to help you prepare for the tests. Bookstores sell study guides. There are also commercial test-preparation courses, which typically cost several hundred dollars.

Steady learning is the best way to prepare for the SAT or ACT, and it doesn't cost a penny. Work consistently on your core courses—particularly English for the verbal portion of the test, and math. Vocabulary and reading comprehension are big parts of the verbal portion, so by reading (even if it's the sports section in your local newspaper) you prepare yourself to do well on the college admissions tests.

Coping with Learning Disabilities

If you suspect that you have a learning disability—such as dyslexia or Attention Deficit Disorder (ADD)—it's important to be assessed by a qualified psychologist or learning specialist. Your school is legally required to accommodate learning-disabled students to help level the playing field in doing course work. The SAT and ACT tests also provide accommodations, such as additional time to take the exams.

If you're receiving accommodations for a learning disability, contact the NCAA to be sure that your grades and scores will be accepted for the purposes of athletic eligibility. The NCAA is skeptical about athletes who fail to meet minimum eligibility requirements and then suddenly discover they have a learning disability. So if you are an athlete who may have a genuine learning disability, it's doubly important to be assessed early.

The NCAA Is Not the Only Game in Town

Scottie Pippen played basketball at the University of Central Arkansas for four years before becoming a top pick in the NBA draft. "So what?" you ask. At the time, Central Arkansas was not a member of the NCAA. It was part of the National Association of Intercollegiate Athletics (NAIA). About 350 four-year colleges and universities throughout the United States and Canada belong to the NAIA. More than 57,000 male and female athletes compete each year for 23 national championships in 13 sports.

Even though the media may give the impression that the NCAA has a monopoly on college sports, that's just not the case. In addition to the NAIA schools, 45,000 athletes at 530 two-year colleges compete in intercollegiate athletic programs under the auspices of the National Junior College Athletic Association (NJCAA). And there are other national associations, such as the National Christian College Athletic Association (NCCAA) and the National Small College Athletic Association (NSCAA). Your choices for getting a college education while continuing your sport extend well beyond the schools in the NCAA.

NAIA Eligibility Requirements

If you are considering attending an NAIA school, read their publication, *Guide for the College-Bound Student*. It includes information on eligibility regulations, financial assistance policies, and recruitment policies. Get their *Guide for Students Transferring from Two-Year Institutions*, if that situation applies to you. Both publications are available by Web, mail, or phone request (see appendix 3).

The NAIA is not burdened by billion-dollar TV deals. Depending on what you're looking for, this is a loss or a blessing. The NAIA does not have the income to support a huge bureaucracy, resulting in less red tape for athletes, high schools, and colleges. For example, there is no Initial-Eligibility Clearinghouse or its equivalent.

In some ways it is easier to be eligible to play your sport at an NAIA college. Entering freshmen must meet two of the following three requirements:

1. A minimum of 18 on the ACT or 860 on the SAT. Unlike the NCAA rules, there is no sliding scale that allows eligibility with a lower ACT or SAT score for athletes with higher grade point averages. Tests must be taken on a national testing date. Scores must be achieved on a single test date. This differs from the NCAA requirement, which permits combining a verbal score from one date with a math score from another.

2. A minimum overall high school grade point average of 2.0 on a 4.0 scale.

3. Graduate in the top half of your high school graduating class.

If you meet the second and third requirements, you can be eligible without taking the ACT or SAT.

Two-Year Colleges and the NJCAA

Accredited junior colleges or community colleges, also known as two-year colleges, offer Associate Degrees in a number of subjects; they also prepare students to transfer to four-year colleges. In some cases, athletic scholarships are available.

Community colleges benefit students who cannot meet the admissions requirements or financial demands of a four-year college. Or perhaps you can get into a four-year college and you want to play

Division I sports, but you're not yet good enough athletically. You might go to a two-year college to further develop your athletic skills, especially if you started your sport late in your high school career.

Information from the NJCAA, which governs junior college sports, is available at their Web site. Their pamphlet *Information for a Prospective NJCAA Student-Athlete* is available by Web, phone, or mail request (see appendix 3).

Entering a community college can be easy. The only requirement is often graduation from high school, or just a minimum age of 18. Students who earn an associate degree can transfer to a four-year college if they meet its academic requirements. Athletes who have qualified through the Initial-Eligibility Clearinghouse based on their high school records can transfer and play after one year.

The NCAA annually publishes a pamphlet entitled *NCAA Transfer Guide* to help athletes who want to transfer from two-year colleges to four-year colleges. You can order the transfer guide by calling the NCAA Hotline (see appendix 3). But let us warn you: you may find mastering differential calculus easier than following the text and charts in the guide.

When you start high school, why not set your sights on getting into a good four-year college? If you make that your goal, it's more likely that you'll push yourself to do the work necessary to gain entrance. If you encounter problems along the way, you can fall back on the community college option, which gives you a second chance for admission to a four-year college.

National Christian College Athletic Association (NCCAA)

The NCCAA provides another opportunity to play sports at the college level. It has a membership of 110 colleges and universities with over 12,000 student-athletes. The organization's mission is to "provide intercollegiate athletics with a Christian perspective." Their eligibility requirements are the same as the NAIA's. You can get information from the NCCAA by Web, phone, or mail request (see appendix 3).

National Small College Athletic Association (NSCAA)

The NSCAA governs sports at 47 colleges, each with an enrollment of under 1,000 students. Information from NSCAA is available from their Web site or by mail (see appendix 3).

Halftime

by Ann Meyers Drysdale

I come from a family of eleven kids. Basketball, baseball, football, and track were as natural in our family as eating and sleeping. Our father, who had played basketball at Marquette University, loved sports and was always teaching us something: how to dribble, serve a tennis ball, high jump, swim. My sister Patty, the first child and an athlete and family leader, also helped create this wonderful, confidence-building environment. I tried to emulate my brother Dave, who is two years older than me, both as a basketball player (he played in the NBA) and as a person (he's a really good guy). We were all competitive. With eleven children in one household, what else could you be? Sports showed us that teamwork led to success. The funny thing was that to compete you had to cooperate.

We also learned to play by the rules. No way were your brothers and sisters going to let you cheat. Losing was bad, but you could feel good about how you played, and you could come back and win the next day. We learned to tell the truth and to respect ourselves and our opponents. To get better you had to work, especially when your older brothers and sisters were bigger, stronger, and faster. The same thing was true in the classroom: to do well, you had to crack the books, not look for a way to get by with doing the minimum.

Our mom, who is generous and giving, ran an open house. We'd bring friends home with us—often whole teams. Many of our friends knew that if you needed an adult to listen and help you figure things out, our mom was there for you. And she'd feed you too.

Our parents were not pushovers. Each of us had chores to do: dust, vacuum, wash cars, pull weeds, put laundry away. We'd go out and play until it was dark, but our homework had to be done first.

Sports and Strong Values

Teamwork, healthy competition, and respect carried over from sports to the rest of our family life. It turns out that what was true for our family is true for the larger society. Drug and alcohol abuse and dropping out are huge problems in high schools today. As a group, young athletes, male and female, do better than other students, despite the publicity when an individual athlete messes up. According to a published study, girls participating in sports have higher self-esteem, are 92 percent less likely to be involved with drugs, are 80 percent less likely to have unwanted pregnancies, and are three times more likely to graduate from high school.

My sisters and I realize now that we were unusual for the 1960s and 1970s, before the upsurge in girls' and women's athletics. People probably called us tomboys, but our dad and our five brothers saw us as fellow athletes. They just wanted to choose up sides and play ball. When I was in elementary school I ran track, which was the only organized sport available to girls in our area. Now, Title IX has been instrumental in opening the way for millions of girls to grow physically, mentally, and emotionally through sports.

When we played organized sports, our parents and brothers and sisters were a big group of fans. My brother David played basketball for Coach John Wooden at UCLA. I arrived at UCLA in 1975, when David was a senior and had played on two NCAA championship teams. He went on to play in the NBA for five years. I was lucky enough to become close to Coach Wooden—or "Papa," as I still call him. I think a lot about Papa's definition of success, and I try to teach it to my children. Success is doing your best to become the best you are capable of becoming. This definition doesn't say anything about wins and losses, fame, or money, yet it led Coach Wooden to ten NCAA Championships. Almost every one of Papa's players graduated and went on to live a useful, rewarding life.

Sports Creates Communities

Kenny Washington, an outstanding player for Papa, was my freshman coach at UCLA. When classes were over for the day, I'd sit in Pauley Pavilion, watch Papa's practices, and do my homework. Then we'd practice, using the same drills. In my senior year, my coach was Billie Moore. My sister Patty had played on Coach Moore's national championship team in 1970 at Cal State Fullerton. Billie Moore coached our Olympic Team to a silver medal in 1976, and led our UCLA team to the National Championship in 1978.

Many people looked at me—a female athlete in the 1970s—as if I had come out of nowhere. I didn't see it that way, because of my family background and because I read. Books were big in my life. In the third grade I read about multisport legend Babe Didrikson and track great Wilma Rudolph and thought, I want to be like them. There was discrimination against women in sports, but some women overcame it. Athletes today who complain about the lack of female role models would be better off going to the library and finding them.

In the spring of 1978 I was drafted by the Houston Angels of the newly formed Women's Basketball League (WBL). But I needed more credits to graduate. I had used up my college eligibility, and playing in the first year of women's professional basketball tempted me. Nevertheless, I took the advice of people who cared about me, stayed at UCLA, and graduated. That turned out to be more important than I realized at the time. In my senior year I took a class in broadcasting from a great teacher, Art Freidman. His class opened my eyes to the possibility of a career in broadcasting. There were already a few female sports broadcasters. One of them was Donna de Varona, who had been an Olympic swimmer.

The Indiana Pacers signed me as a free agent and gave me a tryout. I didn't make the team (wouldn't that have been something?), but they hired me as a broadcaster, and I did about 12 Pacer games. I was only 24, and I wanted to continue as an athlete. The Pacers agreed to release me from my contract so I could play in the WBL for the New Jersey Gems. Except for that brief interlude, I've been a sports broadcaster for 18 years. In 1997 I was asked to play in the WNBA [Women's National Basketball Association]. It's great to still be thought of as an athlete, but I'm the mother of three young children and I did not want to commit to that degree of traveling. As a broadcaster of WNBA games, I can keep my commitments to my kids and still enjoy being part of women's professional basketball.

The Legacy of Don Drysdale

I've had a great life, but like everyone else, I've had my share of adversity. In 1983, my younger sister Kelly, who had been a Little League star and went to Pepperdine University on a basketball scholarship, was killed in a car accident. It was painful for our family to deal with this loss, but it's an article of faith with us that no matter how unfair or even tragic life is, we pick ourselves up and go on.

Ten years later my husband, Don Drysdale, a broadcaster for the Los Angeles Dodgers, went with the team to Montreal. He died there of a heart attack on July 3, 1993. We had been married for seven years, and we had three small children. After Don's death, I cried a lot—for a long time. An outpouring of support from my family and my sports family, and the need to be there for our kids, helped pull me through.

People sometimes ask me for advice on dealing with tragedy. I don't think there is any one right way. Each individual has to find a way that works for them. We all need support, whether it's from family, friends, or organized support groups. I am very conscious that the time Don and I had together was precious. When I am together with my kids, family, and friends, I remind myself just how precious these moments are and that we should never take each other for granted.

One of the qualities I most admired about Don was his respect for people. He cared about people, and it had nothing to do with their position in society. He treated everyone with respect, and he wanted to be treated with respect. When Don gave you his word, that meant everything. He was a fierce competitor, yet at the same time he was a good sport. He loved and respected the game of baseball, but he had a sense of perspective. He knew that ultimately it's just a game. Don was a wonderful husband and father, and it is important for me to keep his memory alive. When I teach my kids that learning and growing from sports are more significant than winning championships, I know I'm passing on Don's legacy.

The Dodgers have included us and become part of our extended sports family, which helps my kids know who their Dad was. We'll go to Dodger Stadium and my sons Don Jr. and Darren will tell me, "See ya." They'll go hang out in the broadcast booth and in the clubhouse with the players.

Working Together

No matter what you're doing, even if it's something as intense and competitive as sports, the most important thing in your life is other people. Don't take them for granted. Cherish them. Our athletic careers last a relatively short time, but ties with other people can last a lifetime. When I was young, most of the mistakes I made had something to do with being stubborn and not listening to the people who cared for me—parents, brothers and sisters, teachers, coaches. I usually paid the price. All this has made me a better and smarter person. Everybody has to deal with trial and error in their lives, but what helps most is when you have people who can help you in these situations. Oftentimes it's a matter of reaching out to family and friends and letting them know you value and welcome their advice.

Now that I'm a mother, I see how important it is to take the time to explain things. Sometimes I'm guilty of just telling my kids what to do. When they ask why, I want to say, "Because I told you so." But young people need to understand why. If there really is no time, a better answer would be, "You need to do this now, and I promise I'll explain it later." Then keep your promise. It's so important to spend time with your kids and give them the attention they'd like to have from you, for that moment can never be recaptured.

The sports community has been a source of support, friendship, comfort, and inspiration to me. A-Game.com is an electronic-age extension of this community. This book and the Web site can help you get the most out of sports, school, and life.

Ann Meyers Drysdale is the color analyst for the Women's NCAA Basketball Tournament and the WNBA on NBC. A member of the Basketball Hall of Fame, Ann led the UCLA basketball team to the National Championship in 1978 and was named the outstanding female athlete in the country.

CHAPTER 10

College Athletics 101

If you play sports in college, or if you intend to, you should understand the business side of college athletics. Regardless of the sport you play and the level you're playing at, the business side of sports can affect you.

For example, the "market" for male gymnasts has declined sharply over the past few years. Why? Because in their efforts to achieve equity under Title IX, many colleges—especially those with major football programs—have terminated their men's gymnastic teams. If you're an athlete with the potential of being recruited, you need to understand the sports business to objectively evaluate the words and actions of coaches and others trying to influence you.

Your high school does not offer a course in the business of college athletics, so we have put one together in the next two chapters.

The first lesson in learning about this business is simple: clear away the hype.

Rah Rah Rah!

College presidents often say that the purpose of athletics at their schools is to generate school spirit and to give students the opportunity to be "well rounded," to develop their bodies as well as their minds, to learn competition and teamwork.

Big-time football and basketball programs may very well generate school spirit. They may also contribute to the well-rounded development of some of their players (although some others only seem to develop well-rounded muscles). But why do hundreds of journalists fill newspaper columns and TV screens with debate about which football team is number-one in the nation? And why do some college coaches earn more than college presidents? Are college sports about more than molding character and creating school spirit?

Big-time basketball and football play a huge role in the nation's entertainment, but these sports involve only 2 percent of all college athletes and only a fraction of a percent of all college students. Why do universities sponsor these programs? How do such multimillion-dollar athletic enterprises fit into a university's academic mission? Read on.

The Big Time

College athletics includes many sports. Which is the most important? For you, the answer is simple. The most important sport is the one you participate in.

Now put yourself in the shoes of the president or athletic director of South Coast State University (SCSU). Which sports are most important to you in this role? They are the ones that bring in the big bucks—the big-time, revenue-producing programs such as football and men's basketball. These are college sports you see on TV throughout the United States, and even throughout the world. Football and men's basketball fill stadiums and arenas with paying customers. Women's college basketball has edged onto the TV screen and has also become a revenue producer at some schools.

A college team, whether it's a big-time one or not, may spend money on the following:

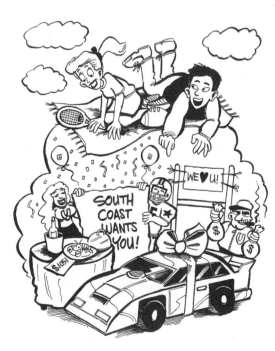

- salaries for head coach and assistant coaches
- salaries for trainers and medical staff
- equipment
- team travel
- public relations
- administrative expenses (office, phone, fax, computer, postage, etc.)
- athletic scholarships
- recruiting (salaries of recruiters, travel, athletes' visits to campus, etc.)

A college team may take in money from the following:

- ticket sales
- radio broadcast rights
- TV broadcast rights
- sale of team-related merchandise
- donations from boosters (we talk about boosters in chapter 11)
- contributions from participants and their families

Now, picture the cross-country team at South Coast. Plenty of money goes out; just check the team expenditure list above. But what funds come in? There are no ticket sales. There is no radio or TV money. SCSU pulls in a lot of money from the sale of merchandise with the college logo and name. But it's the basketball and football teams, with their national TV exposure, that get people to buy SCSU T-shirts, jackets, caps, and mugs. People buy SCSU posters showing football and basketball players. Some SCSU sports other than basketball and football take in more money than the cross-country squad. The hockey and baseball teams gain revenue from ticket sales (but their expenses are also higher than those of the cross-country team).

Most sports programs at SCSU or any other college are like the cross-country team. They spend more than they make, year after year. There are only two sources from which to make up the difference.

- the college's general budget (that is, the same funds that are used to pay for academics, building maintenance, and just about everything else)
- big-time, revenue-producing sports programs

OK, imagine you are still in the shoes of the South Coast president. You are meeting with your Board of Trustees. You want to hire more professors and create new academic programs. But SCSU is a public institution and the state legislature keeps a tight grip on its budget.

Not only that, but you also have to find funds to expand women's sports. Title IX requires that colleges offer equal opportunities in sports to women and men. Do you and the trustees want to finance the men's and women's cross-country teams from the general budget, where the additional salaries for professors could come from? Or do you want to pull the funds from the big-time, revenue-producing sports?

The Need for Victories

What does the football team or the basketball team have to do to pull in as much money as possible? It's simple: win!

Winning can be worth millions of dollars to a college. For example, a win or loss in one game can decide who is invited to a major bowl. The payout for the 1999 Rose Bowl was $13 million per team. Talk about pressure on coaches and athletes.

Winning breeds increased expectations among fans and athletic directors. Big-time athletic departments depend on the financial windfalls of bowl games and NCAA tournament appearances to support all their programs. So even an excellent record, one that might be a success for a team that usually finishes near the bottom, can be a financial setback for a team that is used to winning.

Losing can turn a big-time, revenue-producing program into a bigtime, revenue-losing program. The SCSU football team has huge expenses, including chartering airplanes and overnight stays in luxurious hotels for over a hundred people. Several losing seasons in a row can be a financial disaster for SCSU. Just when the payouts from bowl appearances disappear, boosters' contributions dry up and shoe companies reduce their support. It gets ugly: callers to sports radio shows demand that the coach be fired, and they insult players by name.

As an athlete, it's important to get a feel for the situation you're getting into. Some athletes thrive in the pressure cooker. Others enjoy their sport more when big bucks are not riding on the outcome.

Winning Equals More $$$$

Maybe winning and money shouldn't be tied together, but in reality they are. Why is winning so critical to generating income? Think about the sources of money. People buy more tickets—and they'll pay more for those tickets—to see a winning team. More people watch winning teams on TV, and those are the games TV stations and networks want. They can deliver more viewers to their advertisers, and they can charge their advertisers more. So colleges with winning programs get the most radio and TV money. Football teams that get into bowl games and basketball teams that are invited to the NCAA Tournament make bundles of extra money from tickets, TV, and radio.

One of the biggest sources of funds for college athletic programs is the sale of team-related merchandise: T-shirts, sweatshirts, jackets, caps, posters, pictures, calendars, mugs. People want to identify with winners, so when teams win, sales increase. When a superstar player sets records, sales of merchandise with that player's number also set records. Just take a look at what people are wearing and at what's available in the stores.

How Much Money Are We Talking About?

CBS paid one billion dollars in 1989 for the rights for seven years to broadcast the annual NCAA basketball tournament. But it wasn't enough! As the tournament grew in popularity, the rights increased in value. So CBS held off the competition by negotiating a new agreement with the NCAA. The new agreement, for the eight years from 1995 through 2002, is for $1.725 billion. That's $216 million each year. Along with the rights to broadcast *The Road to the Final Four,* CBS also gets the NCAA baseball finals, the outdoor track championships, women's gymnastics, and the Division II men's basketball final game.

CBS has already signed a contract with the NCAA for 2003 to 2013. This one is for $6 billion—that's $545 million a year. But wait, there's more. There's ESPN, which played such a huge role in making college basketball what it is today. The NCAA agreement with ESPN covers TV rights to the women's basketball tournament and championship matches in a number of other sports. Most of the millions from these contracts goes to the NCAA member colleges through their athletic conferences.

There's still more TV revenue, from all the regular season football games, the bowl games, and the regular season men's and women's basketball games. College sports are also shown on ABC, NBC, and on hundreds of cable channels. But it doesn't stop there. Internet rights to the Final Four and other NCAA hot properties bring in additional—and ever growing—millions.

More revenue is generated from the people who fill the football stadiums, the 40,000, 50,000, or even 100,000 spectators, and from the crowds of 10,000 to 20,000 who pay their way into arenas to watch college basketball night after night. And that's just the ticket revenue.

In 1996, colleges collected royalties on over $2.5 billion in sales of sports-related licensed merchandise. Carl Watson, South Coast's shooting guard, is college basketball's premier player. NBA superscout Buddy Lee describes Carl as "Kobe Bryant—but with a better jump shot." SCSU generates huge revenues from apparel bearing Watson's number, 4. Carl's jersey was the second biggest money maker among all licensed sports apparel—professional and college. Only Kobe Bryant sold more jerseys. But unlike Kobe, Carl could not receive a penny from those sales.

What Makes Coaches Tick?

There's pressure on Babe Steele, SCSU's head basketball coach, to continue winning so the big bucks keep rolling in. If SCSU doesn't win, the trustees, the president, the athletic director, and the boosters will be disappointed. After a few losing years, the athletic director is probably not going to say, "That's OK, Babe. We know your program is molding fine young men. It would be nice if you could win some games, but keep up the good work." He is more likely to say, "Good luck in your next job."

Keeping his job is important to Coach Steele. He and the head football coach are the highest paid employees at SCSU. Coach Steele makes more than his bosses: the athletic director, the college president, and the governor of the state—combined. His base salary alone is $500,000, from a fund supplied by the boosters. In addition, he has a $300,000 consulting contract with Mercury Shoes. The SCSU Marauders wear Merx, which puts the company logo on TV. Coach Steele makes another $200,000 per year from product endorsements, his weekly local TV show, fees for speeches, and the basketball summer camp he conducts at SCSU. That adds up to $1 million a year.

If Coach Steele keeps winning, he can step up to even more income, perhaps to a coaching job in the NBA. If he loses, it can be a big step down. It's not just the money. His kids are happy in the local high school, his wife has a good job and doesn't want to move, and he likes the college and the staff he has put together. After winning the National Championship last year, Coach Steele is treated like a god. If he starts losing, he is demoted from that heavenly position. In fact, the community leaders will tell him to go to the opposite location.

Money Isn't Everything

Coaches in other sports are often under similar pressures. While the biggest money is in basketball and football, winning in any sport can result in advancing to a better job, running a summer camp, coaching in the Olympics, getting endorsement deals, consulting contracts, speaking engagements, and opportunities to write articles and books.

For many coaches, money isn't the main consideration. Most coaches are former athletes. They are competitors who enjoy winning and seeing their athletes win. Winning is fun. Of course, many coaches are believers in Coach Wooden's doctrine that winning means giving your all, regardless of the score. Coach Steele gets upset after a victory if his team played poorly and praises his players after a defeat if they played well.

But the college president is looking for victories. When it comes to squeezing more money out of the boosters, it is victories that count, not effort. So Coach Steele needs the team to win. Of course, he's playing against teams whose coaches are also driven to win. They can't all win. Every time SCSU wins, the other team loses. There will be only one champion in the conference. Over 300 men's Division I basketball teams compete for the NCAA championship. Only 36 football teams will go to bowl games, and half of them will lose.

"Play Here and I'll Make You the Next Michael Jordan"

What does a coach do to win? Two things: recruit the best athletes, and coach them as well as possible.

Which is more important? Everyone agrees that no coach, no matter how great, can win without "the horses." If the opponents' linemen are bigger, stronger, and faster, SCSU probably won't win many football games. If the starting five on opposing basketball teams average three inches taller than SCSU's starting five, and they play just as well, Coach Steele will probably have a losing season.

Coach Steele and his recruiting staff are competing for the best high school players. What will they do to get them? Just yesterday, a prospect told Coach Steele that a recruiter from rival North Coast State University (NCSU) said, "We'll make you the focal point of our offense and showcase you for the NBA." Coach Steele believes the last thing this athlete needs is another boost to his ego, which has been inflated by years of adulation. He wants to tell him, "You're not as good as they've built you up to be. You have a lot of potential, but if you don't work hard you're going to be a bust." Coach Steele wants to say that, but does he take the risk of losing the prospect? Some athletes see it as a sign of respect when a recruiter tells it like it is. But maybe this kid isn't one of those. Should that affect the coach's decision?

The word is that NCSU brings in athletes who don't belong academically and somehow keeps them eligible. There are rumors about cash payments, assignments completed by other students, and SATs taken by ringers. But among the general public, NCSU's reputation is still good.

Coach Steele hates this, because it is not in the athletes' best interest. Does he have to get into this gutter anyway? Can he win if he doesn't? Stay tuned.

A Recruiter Is in Your House

When a recruiter comes to see you, will he or she tell it like it is? Or will he tell you what you want to hear? Do you think he might stress the benefits of his program and omit the drawbacks? For example, he might tell you about the great uniforms and the large crowds, and he might not tell you that the school is under investigation by the NCAA and may face suspension from postseason play for the next two years. The recruiter is out to sell a program: that's his job. Selecting a college that meets your needs is your job.

CHAPTER 11

Other Players in the Recruiting Game

The previous chapter on the business of college athletics gave you the big picture. More details will help you color that picture in. You need to learn about the other players who get involved in the recruiting game.

We've talked about what motivates coaches. In this chapter, we add a few words about the role of assistant coaches, boosters, high school coaches, and "street agents." Let's also consider another group of involved people: your parents, your brothers and sisters, your friends, and you.

Assistant Coaches

Assistant coaches have the same basic motivation as head coaches. They want to create a winning program, for that is their ticket to keeping their jobs and advancing their careers.

Big-time football, basketball, and some other programs have staff members whose title is assistant coach; but their main job is recruiting, not coaching. These assistants locate potential recruits in junior high school or early in their high school careers.

NCAA regulations prohibit Division I coaches or assistant coaches from contacting you before July 1 following your junior year in high school. In football, coaches are allowed to call you once during May of your junior year, but not again until the following September 1. They can come to high school practices or games; they can watch you; but they are not allowed to talk to you in person, or by phone, or write to you. Somehow they manage to make it known they are interested in you. The assistant coaches assigned to recruiting want to build relationships with athletes and help sell their programs.

The head coach sets the tone for every program, determines who plays, and defines the program's attitude toward academics. So when you evaluate a program, you should place a lot of weight on the character, personality, and approach of the head coach.

In some sports, an athlete spends a lot of time with one assistant coach. Football has more assistant coaches than any other sport; there are offensive and defensive coordinators, special teams coaches, quarterback coaches, line coaches, and more. If you're going to be under the direct supervision of an assistant coach, evaluate that coach as well as the head coach.

Boosters

Boosters are well-to-do people who like to be involved with a team. They contribute money, goods, or services to their teams. Some boosters (but not all) are graduates of the college whose team they support.

Some boosters like to know who is being recruited, and they may act independently of the coach. NCAA regulations limit the extent to which boosters can be involved in recruiting (see the *NCAA Guide for the College-Bound Student-Athlete*). But some people simply define themselves as "friends of the program" and get around the rules by not registering as boosters.

In Division I (according to NCAA regulations) boosters are prohibited from contacting potential recruits. In Division II, boosters can write to you or call you after September 1 of your junior year in high school, but they may not contact you in person. Division III boosters can contact you in person after your junior year.

An exception to this ban, according to the NCAA, is if the contact is considered "part of a college's regular admissions program for all prospective students, including nonathletes." But how many boosters do you suppose are out pursuing the next Albert Einstein?

High School Coaches

High school coaches are in a position to influence college selection, for these reasons.

• They have a close relationship with their athletes.
• They may have influence with an athlete's parents.

- Contacts between athletes and college coaches are limited by the NCAA; the high school coach is there every day.

Many high school coaches love their athletes and truly have their best interests at heart. They've been through the recruiting process many times, and they help put limits on recruiters so that athletes can focus on their senior year. Your coach may therefore be an excellent source of advice for you and your parents.

However, you've got to follow the don't-believe-everything-you-hear rule. Even a high school coach with the best intentions may have incomplete information. Or he or she may be biased or may have something to gain from leading you toward one college over another. Steering an athlete toward a college might help a high school coach land consideration for a college job, a summer camp coaching assignment, or some other reward.

Street Agents

People don't identify themselves as *street agents,* which is not a flattering term. Street agents act as go-betweens. They have unofficial relationships with colleges and with high school athletes. Street agents closely follow high school sports, regardless of what else they may do for a living. They may be coaches in summer leagues, AAU coaches, executives of athletic shoe companies, business people, professionals, or factory workers; or they may have no visible means of support. Street agents are likely to have ulterior motives for recommending a college. Be sure to carefully measure the college a street agent recommends against the picture of your ideal school.

Parents

We'll use the word *parent* (or *parents*) to stand for your mother, your father, or anyone else who is acting as your parent. Your parents know you well and understand your strengths and weaknesses. They can help you big time when it comes to selecting a college. But to take advantage of their help, you've got to be open with your parents about what you are looking for in a college.

Listen to your parents' advice, but test it. Ask why. Do they want you to go to a particular college because they were impressed by the coach, or because they have really thought about why it's the best school for you? Are they giving too much weight to a college because it's the one they went to? Are they ruling out colleges that are far away because they can't bear to part with their son or daughter? Or are they ruling out colleges close by?! Do they understand your ideal picture of a college? Have you told them?

One thing your parents may be able to do well is to act as a buffer between you and a recruiter. You may be more comfortable if your parents ask some of the tough questions.

Older Brothers, Sisters, and Friends

If you are fortunate enough to have an older sibling or friend who is selecting a college, you can learn by watching that process. Follow up by talking to him or her about how the college worked out. If your relative or friend is an athlete, fine. If not, better yet. You'll learn how to select a school for academic and social reasons.

Apply your sibling's or friend's experience to your needs. What's right for him or her may not be right for you.

Teammates

Talking over your choices with your teammates can be valuable. Some of them will be selecting colleges at the same time, so you can compare notes and toss ideas around. That's a big plus. Try not to jump to a conclusion based on something a friend says: it may be only one part of a complex picture. You might end up changing your mind from day to day as other parts of the picture jump into focus. If a close friend has a strong opinion, consider it carefully, but don't feel you have to accept it.

You

You're the most important player in the recruiting game because it's your life. When all is said and done, the decision about where to spend the next four years is up to you. You may be limited by what schools will accept you. But that's based largely on what you accomplish athletically and academically in high school.

CHAPTER 12

How to Market Yourself

To successfully market yourself, you have to have a self that's marketable. If you've made yourself the best athlete you can be, studied hard, and lived responsibly, chances are there are college coaches who want you. But they can't want you unless they know you. Marketing means putting yourself in front of them.

For a small percentage of high school athletes, that's not a problem. Coaches are flooding their mailboxes and making their phones ring off the hook. These elite athletes have to cope with too many recruiters rather than too few. The next chapter deals with the special difficulties of that situation, but it's also full of information useful to every athlete. This chapter is mainly for the vast majority of high school athletes who are not pursued by college coaches.

Recruit Your Coach

Most coaches don't have the time or the money to comb the marketplace for athletes. An upstate New York soccer coach doesn't have the recruiting budget to scout Southern California. So if coaches can't recruit you, you have to recruit them.

This effort can result in an athletic scholarship, but even if it doesn't, a coach in your corner can help you be admitted to the college of your choice. Remember, college admission is the prerequisite to collecting any kind of financial aid.

Here are the steps to follow in recruiting a coach.

Make a List of Potential Schools

Step one in recruiting a coach is to select a group of colleges you might want to attend, based on their academic, athletic, and social characteristics. In chapter 7, we covered the search for the right school, and we presented one driving principle of your search: pick schools you would like even if there were no sports.

Cast your net wide. Come up with a preliminary list of at least 25 schools. Ask everybody you know, and everybody they know, for suggestions and introductions. Search the Internet for colleges that field teams in your sport (A-Game.com has links to help you do that).

Pare Your List Down

Once you've built up your initial list, the next step is to carve it down. Contact the coaches, by e-mail or snail mail. Some programs have forms for this purpose. Tell the coach that you are interested in playing on his or her team. Briefly, and objectively, describe your athletic and academic accomplishments. Include your height and weight. If articles have been written about your performance, you may want to include one or two. Include your team's schedule if you think the coach might want to scout you. Your goal at this stage is not to make the sale but to find out if the coach wants to know more.

Follow Up Aggressively

Some coaches will not respond to your letter, but don't assume this is because they have studied your letter and have already decided against you. Their agenda is not your agenda; they have dozens of other tasks to field. For example, you may be a state medallist in the shot put and have a 4.0 grade point average, but if a coach is busy preparing her team for the tournament, she may have your letter on a stack of unopened mail.

To avoid missing out on a program that may be a great fit for you, follow up aggressively. In most cases, the best way to follow up is by phone or e-mail.

Don't Be Intimidated

Many teenagers would rather write a ten-page paper than call an adult they don't know. But coaches have told us they are impressed by athletes who have the guts to call. Mostly they hear from parents or recruiting services. When you call, it's the coach's first indication that you're a go-getter with a strong desire to succeed. By talking directly to the coach, you begin to build a relationship. Use the phone call to learn more about the coach and the team.

Close In

Based on the responses to your initial letters and to your follow-up, make a list of about six schools that have shown interest. Now you are going for the sale. Send them a compelling package to show them why they need you. Your package should include these basic elements.

- an explanation of how you will contribute to the team
- a summary of your athletic achievements
- a description of your academic record

Include a brief cover letter. List your height, weight, and your athletic and academic qualifications on a separate sheet. Even if you have already sent this information, send it again. Don't make the coach search for your first letter. You might also send photos of yourself participating in your sport, photocopies of clippings about your performance, and a videotape showing you in competition, if that's appropriate to your sport.

The videotape should not be a highlight reel. A coach wants to evaluate your complete game. You should appear at the beginning of the tape to introduce yourself. When the tape shows you in competition, be sure it's easy for viewers to identify you. If you're in a team sport, you can have your name and number appear at the bottom of the frame. If you play an individual sport and there are other athletes in the frame (for example in swimming or track), consider having an arrow point to you. Appear again at the end of the tape, reintroduce yourself, and thank the coach for watching. Include your phone number and e-mail address, which should also be written on the cassette label and the box.

Do your homework on the teams you are contacting. When you're exchanging e-mail or letters with the coach, or talking on the phone, try to accumulate information about the team. Then include something in each cover letter about why your contribution would be valuable to that particular team. For example, you could point out that their starter and backup in your position are graduating seniors. Or that your abilities fit in with the coach's style of play. Your package will stand out from other packages that are not customized. A buyer appreciates a seller who considers his or her particular needs.

All your written material should be typed, and you should check for spelling, grammar, and appearance before it goes out the door. Two sets of eyes are better than one; ask a parent or teacher to proofread. One of the worst mistakes you can make is to show carelessness by misspelling the coach's name or the name of the college. You are competing for a scholarship, so pay attention to every detail that can help you win. This professional approach will serve you throughout your life—whether you are applying for a job or trying to sell people on your ideas.

Online Recruiting

A number of companies are attempting to bring athletes and coaches together on the Internet. As of this moment, the industry leader appears to be LevelEdge.com. Online recruitment is an idea whose time undoubtedly will come. You have nothing to lose by listing yourself on LevelEdge, or on other sites where you can post your data for

---

Should You Hire a Recruiting Agency?

Finding athletic scholarships has become big business, and there has been an explosion in the number of companies selling this service to athletes and their families.

Athletes who can least afford to hire these agencies are the athletes who most need scholarships. Recruiting agencies generally charge between $100 and $1,500, depending on what they say they are going to do. The agencies justify their fees by comparing them to the greater value of an athletic scholarship. There are two problems with this comparison.

1. You pay up front, whether you get a scholarship or not.
2. You might have been able to get the scholarship yourself.

Recruiting agencies say that coaches are more likely to believe their estimates of your ability than your own. According to the agencies, coaches know that the agencies will not inflate an athlete's talent, because the reputation of the agency would be at risk.

If you prepare your own package, you can add this objectivity by asking a rival coach to write a recommendation. The college coach will know that a coach from a rival high school has no personal stake in recommending you.

If you can put together a recruiting package on your own, we recommend that you do so. Coaches tell us they are more impressed by do-it-yourself efforts than by commercially produced packages.

---

free. But don't rely on the Internet as your primary method of attracting the attention of coaches. Online recruitment has not yet caught on with most coaches.

Advanced Market Research

Successful businesses do market research to help them determine where and how to sell their products and services. When you asked people for suggestions about where you would have the best chance to play your sport, you were conducting your own market research. The tables in this chapter that chart sports participation and scholarship limits (see pages 108–111) will help you learn more about the market for your athletic services in NCAA schools.

For example, let's say you are a male fencer seeking a Division III program. You know of four programs, but the table tells you there are a total of 15 Division III fencing teams. Now you know there are 11 more Division III colleges out there where you could fence. A-Game.com is a good place to search for additional programs.

In addition to the number of teams in each division in each sport, the table tells you the size of an average team in that sport and the maximum number of scholarships permitted by the NCAA. Knowing how many teams there are and their average size helps you estimate your chances of playing. Knowing the maximum number of scholarships permitted helps you determine your odds of getting one. The next step is to ask a coach the number his or her program actually awards.

There are many ways to slice, dice, and use this information. Consider these statistics an important tool to use in your search.

Row, Row, Row Your Boat Gently to the Bank

When comparing men's and women's statistics, you may find some data that you don't understand. For example, the women's table reveals that there are 75 Division I women's rowing (crew) programs. The average squad size is 55, and each one can award up to twenty scholarships. You might not picture Iowa and Kansas as flowing with rivers, but the University of Iowa and the University of Kansas are among the schools with women's crew.

The number of Division I men's rowing programs is a big, round zero. This is particularly intriguing because there are men's rowing programs at many of these colleges; they are just not under the NCAA umbrella and do not award scholarships. Why is this? With gender equity required by Title IX, colleges must do something to balance the 85 (Division I-A) or 63 (Division I-AA) football scholarships. Twenty rowing scholarships for women and zero for men is part of the solution.

Learn What Your Odds Are

Let's go back to women's rowing. You know that there are 1,500 full scholarships available in Division I women's rowing, and that up to 4,125 athletes (75 teams **x** 55 athletes/team) can get at least a portion of one. Almost no public high schools have rowing programs. There-fore if you are a strong, well-coordinated female athlete, you have an excellent chance of earning an athletic scholar-ship as a rower. If you are a petite female with a command-ing voice and a sure hand, you might land one of these scholarships as a coxswain.

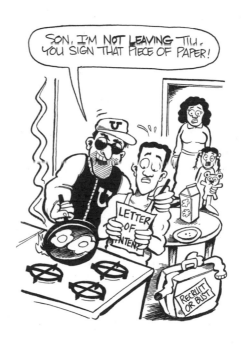

Opportunity in women's rowing is just one nugget that can be mined from the data in the table. For example, if you are a multisport athlete, the table can help you determine which of your sports to focus on in the college selection process. Study the numbers and conduct other market research in your sport.

NCAA Men's Sports Participation and Scholarship Limits

	Division I		
	Teams[3]	Average Squad	Scholarship Limit[4]
Baseball	285	34	11.7
Basketball[5]	321	15	13
Cross-country[7]	300	15	12.6
Fencing[6]	20	17	4.5
Football I-A[5]	114	114	85
I-AA[5]	122	92	63
Golf	283	11	4.5
Gymnastics	23	15	6.3
Ice hockey[5]	55	28	18
Lacrosse	54	40	12.6
Rifle[6]	4	7	3.6
Skiing[6]	12	16	6.3
Soccer	198	27	9.9
Swimming	151	25	9.9
Tennis	276	13	4.5
Track & field[7]	265	32	12.6
Volleyball	23	25	4.5
Water polo	24	25	4.5
Wrestling	91	30	9.9

1. All Division II sports are equivalency; equivalency sports are allowed to divide a full scholarship among more than one student athlete.
2. Division III does not award athletic scholarships.
3. Teams as of 1999–2000.
4. This is the maximum allowed by the NCAA. Many colleges do not have the funds to award them all.
5. Head count sport.

Division II[1]			Division III[2]	
Teams[3]	Average Squad	Scholarship Limit[4]	Teams[3]	Average Squad
232	31	9	343	27
290	14	10	383	17
220	11	12.6	308	13
1	9	4.5	15	14
156	87	36	220	82
180	9	3.6	243	10
1	12	5.4	2	20
11	27	13.5	66	29
32	29	10.8	118	28
0	0	3.6	3	11
8	14	6.3	20	13
168	25	9	359	24
51	17	8.1	179	17
179	10	4.5	312	10
148	26	12.6	233	28
18	14	4.5	40	11
5	19	4.5	15	19
41	25	9	106	22

6. Coed championship sport.
7. Track and cross-country scholarships are divided among 12.6 scholarships total.
Source: NCAA and A-Game.com 2000 survey of 48 college coaches and
administrators.

NCAA Women's Sports Participation and Scholarship Limits

	Division I		
	Teams[3]	Average Squad	Scholarship Limit[4]
Basketball[2,5]	317	14	15
Cross-country[4,7]	316	15	18
Fencing[6]	25	13	5
Field hockey	75	23	12
Golf	190	9.0	6
Gymnastics[2,5]	67	14	12
Ice hockey	25	23.4	18
Lacrosse	69	24.7	12
Rifle[3,6]	10	4.6	??
Rowing (Crew)	75	55	20
Skiing[3,6]	14	16	7
Soccer	262	23.7	12
Softball	238	18.5	12
Squash	7	16	12
Swimming/Diving	180	24.4	14
Sync. Swimming	6	11.3	5
Tennis[2,5]	309	9.3	8
Track[4,7]	277	29.7	18
Volleyball[2,5]	307	13.6	12
Water polo	22	22.3	8

1. All Division II sports are equivalency; equivalency sports are allowed to divide
   a full scholarship among more than one student athlete.
2. Division III does not award athletic scholarships.
3. Teams as of 1999–2000.
4. This is the maximum allowed by the NCAA. Many colleges do not have the
   funds to award them all.

Division II[1]			Division III[2]	
Teams[3]	Average Squad	Scholarship Limit[4]	Teams[3]	Average Squad
287	14	10	414	14
248	10	12.6	332	12
1	7	4.5	20	11
26	23	6.3	144	21
70	8.0	5.4	115	8
7	14	6.0	17	16
2	19	18.0	26	19
23	23	19.9	133	20
0	6	??	2	4
13	27	20	40	34
9	10	6.3	21	11
184	21	9.9	372	21
248	17	7.2	367	17
0	0	9.0	22	13
65	18	8.1	219	19
0	0	5.0	4	13
211	8	6.0	356	10
277	20	12.6	244	21
270	13	8.0	394	14
6	19	8.0	12	17

5. Head count sport.
6. Coed championship sport.
7. Track and cross-country scholarships are divided among 12.6 scholarships total.
Source: NCAA and A-Game.com 2000 survey of 48 college coaches and
   administrators.

CHAPTER 13

Control Your Recruitment

You are a heavily recruited athlete. You've created a picture of the right college for you, using the method we outlined in chapter 7, and you understand the business of recruitment. Now the challenge is to manage the recruitment process so you make the best choice while putting the least pressure on yourself. You want to enjoy your senior year in high school.

Selecting a College Is Like Buying Your First Car

Recruiting in some sports starts as early as the eighth grade. If recruiters have been after you for years, you might think you already know all the answers. Big mistake. You are up against recruiters who have been adults longer than you have been alive. If you try to outsmart them on your own, you are setting yourself up for a loss. The way to win—which means ending up at the right college for you—is to take advantage of the experience of others.

You will probably select a college only once—and that creates a problem. You normally learn by correcting your mistakes. But when selecting a college there's no second chance, so you don't have that luxury.

To compound the problem, college recruiters usually have much more experience and savvy than you do. They've talked to hundreds of potential recruits and they've made dozens of "sales."

The situation is similar to that facing first-time car buyer Maya Edwards, a hockey player at South Coast State University (SCSU). As Maya walks onto the used car lot, she is nervous and unsure of which questions to ask the salesperson. The cars all look attractive, but her eyes land quickly on a red convertible that's out of her budget. She pictures herself pulling up to her friend's house in that sleek car, and Maya soon forgets that she came to buy a pickup truck.

The salesperson recognizes the look in Maya's eyes. The next thing Maya knows, she's driving that red convertible off the lot. "How did that happen?" is what she wonders each month when she writes a check for her car loan; it's what she asks herself as she tries to cram her gear into her car's tiny trunk.

Think Before You Buy

If you were buying a car, what would you do to avoid Maya's mistakes? How does that apply to recruiting?

Ask Questions Until You Get Answers

Maya didn't dig for the truth by asking questions. She could have asked the salesman what the loan's interest would add to the price of the car. She could have asked him if the car was suitable for transporting gear on back roads. The salesman had no reason to volunteer this information. He didn't know her budget or that she wanted to use the car for camping trips.

The salesman could have sold Maya a more suitable car by asking her about her requirements. Maya might then have become a customer for life and recommended the salesperson to her friends. But maybe the salesman didn't know any better, or maybe he was out for the fast buck. Unfortunately, Maya's best interests were sacrificed at the same time.

You may deal with recruiters who operate this way out of ignorance, greed, or just because they're in a hurry. By asking questions until you uncover the truth, you protect your interests. You also protect the recruiter from making the wrong decisions and ending up with athletes who don't fit in with their programs or their colleges.

Control Your Ego

As an athlete, you know that when you compete, you have to concentrate on your goals. Your opponents may talk trash, the crowd may cheer or boo. You have to control your ego to avoid making spur of the moment decisions based on emotions instead of goals.

The salesman used Maya's ego in just that way, and he appealed to her emotions about that red convertible. To protect yourself from a similar situation, you might talk to people who have bought cars before. You might make a list of questions to ask them beforehand. You might bring an experienced car buyer with you to the showroom and postpone a decision until you can consult with your advisor. In that way, you'd be on a more equal basis with the salesperson.

We've blamed overzealous recruiters for many problems. But athletes and their parents are also at fault for not asking enough questions. A recruiter is not doing you a favor by talking to you: he or she believes you may benefit the team. Feel free to ask anything you want. Be open and honest. If you don't understand an answer, keep asking.

A recruiter who is thoughtful about matching his or her program to your needs will welcome your questions. If the recruiter won't give you straight answers or seems tired of your questions, you've discovered something. Do you want to attend a school where the coach is put off by your desire to learn the facts?

Maintain Your Amateur Status

If the NCAA decides you are a professional athlete, you lose your college eligibility. And there's not much of an appeals process.

It's easy to become what the NCAA defines as a professional athlete. For example, you are a pro if you are "paid (in any form) or accept the promise of pay for playing in an athletics contest." Suppose you're on a summer basketball team. The coach—a well-known street agent—pays to fly the team to the beach and treats each player to a shopping spree in a sporting goods store he owns. Presto: You are a pro twice over. Once for the trip; once for the shopping. This type of thing goes on, but you should know that you can lose your college eligibility if you get caught.

Another way you can become a pro before you want to is if you "use your athletics skill for pay in any form (for example, TV commercials, demonstrations)." Or if you "sign a contract or verbally commit with an agent or a professional sports organization." "Also," writes the NCAA, "receiving any benefits or gifts by you, your family or friends from a player agent would jeopardize your college eligibility." Things that are free often have higher price tags than things you pay for. This is especially true in those revenue-producing sports where ulterior motives seem to lurk.

Agents: Strangers Offering Candy

Sometimes agents, their employees, or others who look to benefit from your athletic ability will act as though they are concerned only for your welfare. They just happen to want to be your friend and offer you clothes, money, even a car. Or maybe they have a nice job for your Uncle Harry.

It's tough for high school and college athletes—especially those who are flat broke—to turn down these offers. Before you put your

A Coach and a Ballplayer Both Strike Out

Bonita Lind, a high school softball pitcher in her senior year, has attracted national attention by setting strike-out and shut-out records. Bonita is also an excellent hitter and fielder. She dreams of playing in the Olympics, which will take place when she's a junior in college. Bonita believes that focusing on raising her pitching to a higher level will make her dream a reality. She's considering going to South Coast, which plays in a conference with some of the top softball teams in the country.

Bonita is talking to Meg Rose, the legendary coach of the South Coast women's softball team. South Coast already has a sophomore who is a great pitcher, but the team could use more power at the plate. So Coach Rose wants to put Bonita in the outfield, where her strong arm will help the team. But Bonita doesn't think the outfield is her route to the Olympics.

Bonita asks Coach Rose if she will be able to pitch as a freshman. The Coach replies, "Sure, you'll pitch in some of our games." Meg is thinking that Bonita will be the starting pitcher in about four games, when the team's regular pitcher needs rest. But Bonita thinks "some of our games" means about half of the games—or maybe all of them. Bonita hears it that way because she wants it to be that way. Bonita doesn't request a more specific answer because she doesn't want to seem disrespectful to Meg Rose, who has coached two U.S. Olympic teams and whose books on softball are read all over the world.

Bonita's freshman year arrives and she is in for a disappointment. So is Coach Rose, who didn't expect to have an unhappy player. Bonita is partially responsible for the miscommunication. She should have tried to nail down what the coach meant by "some of our games." Coach Rose didn't even know that Bonita's Olympic hopes were tied to pitching. If Bonita had told the coach of her desire to pitch in the Olympics, the Coach might not have given such a casual answer. In fact, she might have given Bonita the benefit of her experience about the best way for Bonita to make the Olympic team.

There are several lessons you can learn from this story.
- Don't be intimidated (which is easier said than done).
- Make sure you get clear answers to your questions—and ask until you do.
- Let the coach know what is on your mind and why.
- Take advantage of every interview to learn something. For example, why not ask a coach what he or she thinks you should do to improve?

hand out, think about what you are doing. Many athletes violate the NCAA rules and get away with it. But if you are caught, you have to live with the consequences. You risk your college athletic career, a college education, and possibly a pro contract.

Even if you accept gifts from agents or others and you don't get caught, you still lose. In one way or another, you owe something to those who give you money, goods, or favors. They are in it for profit. They give you what for them is chump change, with the intention of eventually collecting on their investment in you. They invest in many athletes, and they profit if only a few of those players become pros. So their risk is spread out, and any one young athlete is expendable. If you get caught, their profits continue. (We talk more about agents in chapter 15.)

How to Manage Recruiters

When Barry Switzer was head football coach at Oklahoma University, he desperately wanted to recruit Billy Sims (who went on to win the 1979 Heisman Trophy). Legend has it that Coach Switzer sent an assistant to Billy's hometown with instructions not to return without Billy. Talk about recruiting pressure! The assistant checked into a nearby motel but spent all his time with Billy and his family. He reportedly even cooked their breakfasts. The assistant was finally able to return home—and keep his job—when, after 68 days, Billy signed.

If you are a top athlete in a sport with big budgets, you will be swamped with letters, phone calls, email, and personal contacts from recruiters. This attention may seem glamorous at first, but it can take too much of your time. You lose effectiveness as a student and as an athlete, and it becomes tough to enjoy high school. Here are some suggestions for dealing with recruiters.

- Limit when you and your parents are available for phone calls. Instruct recruiters, for example, to phone only on Tuesdays and Thursdays from 7 to 9 P.M. If recruiters call at other times, politely explain when they should call.
- Limit whom you want to deal with, what you want to talk about, and how long you want to talk. For example, you can politely tell a coach or assistant coach that you are considering his or her school, but you do not want any calls from boosters and/or calls from anybody just wanting to chat about how well you did in your last game.

- Narrow down the number of colleges you are considering by ruling out those that differ too much from your ideal picture. Once you know a college doesn't have all the features on your must-have list, you can stop wasting time on their letters and phone calls. And you don't need to take time to visit their campuses.

Benefit from Every Phone Call

You should know why you are talking to a particular recruiter at a particular time. If you have already ruled out a college, there's no reason to be on the phone with that school's recruiter at all. If you are still considering a college, your ideal picture is the starting point. How does this college compare? What do you still need to learn to make the comparison? Getting that information should be the goal of your phone call.

If you're like most of us, you'll remember a question you meant to ask just after you hang up. To prevent this, write down the questions that apply to this phone call; check them off as you write down the answers. Keep a box of note cards next to the phone, with a card for each college you are considering. You will be collecting so much information that it will become a jumble unless you write it all down. If you rely on memory, you will become confused about which coach at which college said what. There may also be information you want to bring to the recruiter's attention. Write that down too.

You want to control the phone call, but give the recruiter time to provide information to you. If it's a first contact, listen to his or her whole story, then ask questions. Make sure to find out if the school has all the features on your must-have list and the features you consider to be important.

If you are shy when dealing with adults, this may be hard. But the benefit of getting information that satisfies your needs is enormous, so grit your teeth and ask. Remember that you are in a powerful position. Even if the coach is a legend, he or she can't win without athletes.

After the first contact with a recruiter, listen for new information. For example, the recruiter may tell you that you are now their number-one choice because two athletes have signed elsewhere or that the college's needs have changed in some other way.

You don't have to stay on the phone while the recruiter goes over old ground or asks what your favorite food is. You can politely end the conversation at any time.

You and your parents may want to confer during a phone call.

That's OK, and it's not a sign of weakness. Just tell the recruiter that you want to discuss something with your parents and would he or she mind holding on for a minute.

At any time during a phone call, feel free to ask recruiters to mail you information so that you can study it in detail. If they agree to send the information, see if they do. It's one test of how serious they are about you and about keeping their promises.

Asking for information in writing is a good tactic when you feel that the recruiter is exaggerating. Jonathan Krone's father said that the North Coast State baseball coach "guaranteed" that Jonathan, a star outfielder, would be in the starting lineup as a freshman. Mr. Krone thought that was an extraordinary claim: the college had several outfielders who were not seniors, and they were trying to recruit other top high school players. He asked the coach to put the guarantee in writing. Here's what the coach wrote: "Jonathan will start as a freshman if his performance demonstrates he is most qualified at his position."

Don't Believe the Hype (DBTH)

Recruiters often praise athletes to the skies, treat them to luxurious meals and accommodations, and create hoopla to influence their decisions. A-gamers don't allow this hype to go to their heads: they keep their feet on the ground.

DBTH (Don't Believe the Hype) should be the golden rule of college recruitment. But how do you apply this golden rule? Should you buy a lie detector and hook up every person who tells you how great some college will be for you?

A better tactic is to treat everybody as if they were honest. That way, you don't become cynical and risk cutting yourself off from close ties with good people who care about you.

However, when you treat people as if they were honest, you have to understand that things change. When a coach tells you that you are going to start as a freshman, just add in your mind, "unless someone better is available when the season starts." If a coach says that an NCAA investigation of his school won't lead to sanctions, add "unless additional evidence turns up." "You are the next Michael Jordan" means, "You might be the next Michael Jordan if you develop into a better athlete than the 10,000 other young athletes who are also the next Michael Jordan."

If you're busy figuring out if someone is lying, it's hard to pay attention to what he or she is saying. You get distracted by trying to read facial expressions or body language. Your ego also gets involved. You might end up rejecting a good college because you thought a recruiter lied.

Treating everybody as though they were honest may seem naive. But efforts to detect lies often fail, because the best and most experienced liars come across as sincere. Treating people as honest is actually a more powerful weapon for getting at the truth. To use this method, listen carefully and ask lots of questions. Be like a trial lawyer who asks a lot of questions to discover *the whole truth*.

Negative Recruiting

A recruiter may try to sign you up by knocking the opposition. This negative recruiting tells you nothing about the school the recruiter represents. You may want to listen first, then ask a recruiter from the school under attack to respond to any points that concern you. You should not believe statements made by a recruiter about a competing school without hearing that response. And you are within your rights to cut off the negative comments by telling the recruiter you would prefer to hear about his or her program.

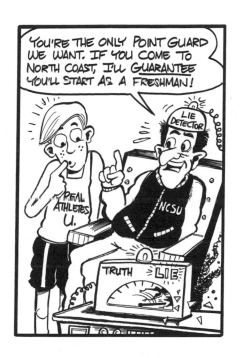

Take Advantage of Home Visits

The NCAA has reduced the number of times recruiters are allowed to visit your home. Therefore, recruiters usually pack the limited time available with all their selling points. Their presentations may include glossy full-color brochures and videotapes worthy of Hollywood.

In the good ol' days of recruiting, coaches gave the same presentation to everyone; it was a cookie-cutter approach to recruiting. Many still give the same presentation, but competition for athletes has led to a practice of customized dog-and-pony shows. The coach finds out what you like and what you don't, and he or she tries to push the right buttons to get you to sign. Whether you're presented with the cookie-cutter version or the customized presentation, ask questions to determine whether the program really meets your needs.

Most of what we said about phone contacts also applies to home visits. Feel free to ask any questions you want. Prepare checklists of those questions. If you have information to present to the recruiter, have notes about that as well. You are both trying to figure out if you, the athletic program, and the college will make a good fit. If the recruiter doesn't know what you are looking for, he or she is flying blind. The best recruiters will probe for this information, but others will just stick with their canned or customized presentations unless you take the lead.

Take nothing for granted. If it isn't clear, be sure to ask the big question, "Are you offering me an athletic scholarship?"

Don't Sign the NLI under the Gun

A recruiter may ask you to sign the NLI (National Letter of Intent) during a home visit. We suggest that you don't do it. Throw away the pen. The dotted line will still be there tomorrow.

Unless you've absolutely decided beforehand, signing during a visit is one of the worst recruiting mistakes you could make.

If you want to commit to a college, why not sign? Especially if the coaches tell you they are considering other athletes and their scholarship offer may be withdrawn?

Here's why. It's possible that the offer may be taken away within a few days, but it's not likely, especially if the coaching staff is committed to you.

It's probable that you will have second thoughts. Take a few days to recover from the pressure. Compare your ideal picture of a college to this college at least one more time.

After your second thoughts, you may decide this college is best for you. That's fine. Having your second thoughts before making your final decision shows maturity. You will feel much better than if you had rushed into a commitment.

Take Advantage of Campus Visits

Did you see the movie *Blue Chips*? In the film, the coach takes three players he is recruiting into a 15,000-seat arena. They stand on the basketball court. The arena is dark, silent, empty. Suddenly spotlights sweep the floor and upbeat music fills the air. The players hear their names announced over the PA system, as though they were starting a game for Western University. What a rush for a 17-year-old high school athlete!

Many programs similarly try to dazzle athletes rather than give them a realistic idea of what it would be like to attend that college. One coach we spoke to warned against getting snowed by, "a campus visit that is a 48-hour magic carpet ride, filled with experiences that will never be part of your normal routine at the university."

A campus visit is a good opportunity to do your homework about a particular school, so make sure you use your time well during those visits. Here are some additional tips.

Talk to the Team

On a campus visit, you will be spending time with the coaching staff and the athletes on the team. It's the best opportunity for you to get a feel for the system and the people. Are you comfortable? Will you fit in? Do you like the way the coach runs practice?

Don't talk only to the stars or the players you are steered toward. Talk to the athletes who don't get as much playing time and to the people you feel will be straight with you (maybe somebody you played with or against in high school). Have private conversations. Introduce yourself and explain that you are thinking of coming to this school next fall. Start with open questions such as, "What has your experience here been like?" or, "Could you tell me what you like and don't like about being here?" These questions are most apt to produce long responses containing lots of information. If you ask a closed question such as, "Do you like it here?" you are likely to get only a yes or a no answer. That kind of answer tells you nothing about why you would like the school. Questions that start with what, why, and how will draw out the most information.

If you meet an athlete who is unhappy with his college experience, it's not necessarily the fault of the program or the coach. See if his case is an isolated incident or if you have spotted a trend. Talk to enough people so you get the full picture.

Get Information That Is Available Only on Campus

Do not waste your time on a campus visit getting information that is available from other sources, such as the school catalog. Before visiting SCSU, Joe Shott told the basketball coach that he wanted to meet some of the communications faculty and sit in on their classes. The coach included these items in Joe's schedule. By thinking ahead, Joe picked up information he could only have gotten from a campus visit—a first-hand impression of the communications department. Joe impressed the basketball coach and the professors. They saw him as a heads-up guy who takes initiative, makes plans, and carries them out.

Campus Visits: Technicalities Can Make or Break You

There are two ways you can visit a college campus: at your expense or at the school's expense. Some colleges have big budgets for financing campus visits, and others don't. The NCAA has complex rules governing college visits. Plan your visits well ahead of time so that you can use the technicalities to your advantage rather than be tripped up by them.

For example, you are limited to visiting no more than five campuses at the colleges' expense. Therefore be sure you go only to colleges you're seriously considering. Make sure your test scores and transcripts are submitted in time to allow a college to pay for your visit.

These are a few of the many rules that govern visits to Division I colleges in the 1999–2000 *NCAA Guide for the College-Bound Student-Athlete*. The rules are different for Divisions II and III, and they may change from year to year.

NCAA Rules for Visits to Division I Colleges

- You can visit a college campus at any time at your expense.
- During your senior year, you can accept no more than one expense-paid (official) visit to a particular campus.
- You may make official visits to no more than five colleges.
- You can't make an official visit unless you have given the college your high school (or college) official academic transcript and a score (it doesn't have to be a qualifying score) from a PSAT, an SAT, a PACT Plus, or an ACT test taken on a national test date under national testing conditions.

Campus Visits: Key Points

Here is a summary of key points to remember when you arrange campus visits.

- Know the NCAA rules.
- Schedule visits way ahead of time.
- Submit your transcripts and test scores in advance.

- Visit only colleges you are seriously considering.
- Learn about the college before your trip. Use your visit to get information that's not available off campus.
- Look for the reality beneath the glitter.
- Don't accept or reject an offer of an athletic scholarship during the visit. Go home and think about it first.

National Letter of Intent

What is the National Letter of Intent (NLI)? The name contains three clues.

National: The same letter is used by most NCAA colleges in the United States.

Letter: It is a letter—actually a complex contract—that you sign to accept an athletic scholarship.

Intent: The National Letter of Intent binds you to a particular college. They don't grant this exemption in the NLI, but most lawyers agree that you can get out of it in the event of your own death. Otherwise, you are stuck even if you change your mind. In the NLI you agree that if you go to another college instead, you cannot play for two years and you will have only two years of eligibility remaining. The letter refers to this as a "basic penalty," but it sounds more like cruel and unusual punishment. That's one more reason why it's so important to be thorough about selecting the right college.

What's Good about the NLI?

The NLI protects colleges from each other, and it protects you from continued recruiting pressures after you make a decision. Once you've signed with one school, other colleges will stop banging on your door.

Without the NLI, there would be no penalty against an athlete who accepted an athletic scholarship and then continued to shop around to other colleges. A college would make a commitment to an athlete but would receive no commitment from the athlete in return.

What's Bad about the NLI?

You select a college because of what it has to offer, and you sign the NLI with that college. Then things change at the college: the features that attracted you are no longer there.

You're stuck.

What might change? The coach, for example, could leave. We hope you won't select a college based only—or even mainly—on the coach, even though, for any athlete, the coach is an important part of the equation. But let's say you pick the coach that's right for you. Suddenly, he or she is gone from that school. If the new coach has an approach that you don't like, that's too bad.

Many athletes have signed the NLI, only to be burned when a coach departs. The people who administer the NLI have responded by emphasizing that even if the coach leaves, you stay. They've put a border around NLI Article 19, so that you can't miss it. Here it is.

> *19. If Coach Leaves. I understand that I have signed this NLI with the institution and not for a particular sport or individual. For example, if the coach leaves the institution or the sports program, I remain bound by the provisions of the NLI.*

What other changes at the college might cause you to regret signing the NLI? The school might be found guilty of violating NCAA rules and become banned from postseason play. The coach might have recruited another phenom at your position, even though he or she promised not to. There could also be cuts in the academic department that attracted you.

Sign Early or Late?

You can sign the NLI only at designated times during your senior year in high school or your final year in junior college. Basketball has a one-week early signing period in November and a late signing period from early-April to mid-May. Football has one signing period, from early February to early April. Many other sports have November early signing periods and late signing periods from mid-April through July. Still others have just one signing period, from early February through July. Each year's NCAA guide publishes the exact signing dates for all sports. During the late signing period, the offer is considered withdrawn if you don't sign the letter within 14 days of the date it was issued.

When to sign the National Letter of Intent is a tactical decision you face in the recruiting process. Should you sign early or late? If you sign late, should you sign at the beginning of the period, in April, or at the end, in July?

Reasons to Sign Early

There are three reasons for accepting an offer right away and signing the NLI early.

1. You are certain that this is the college for you.

2. You don't want to risk losing the scholarship by not accepting it.

3. You want to end the recruiting pressure and enjoy the rest of your senior year in high school or your final year in a two-year college.

Reasons to Wait

There are three reasons for waiting to sign the NLI.

1. The November early signing period is almost a year before you will go to college. You don't want to be locked in if things change at the college, or if your needs change.

2. You think there's a good chance you'll get an offer from a college you would prefer to attend.

3. You can tolerate the recruiting pressure. It doesn't prevent you from enjoying athletics, doing your schoolwork, or preparing for your college entrance exams.

Beware of Verbal Commitments during Campus Visits

Recruiters are not permitted to ask you to sign the NLI during a campus visit. Instead, they may ask you to make a verbal commitment to their program. We suggest that you avoid doing that. Once you have given your word, you want to keep it. But then what do you do if you have second thoughts?

If you see or hear things during a visit that convince you not to attend the school, don't immediately say no. After more thought, you may decide that the college looks pretty good after all. You could call back and say you changed your mind (coaches do understand that young people change their minds), but why put yourself under that pressure in the first place.

So how should you respond during a visit if a coach asks you to commit? Express your appreciation for the confidence the coach has shown in you and tell the coach you want to think about it for a few days.

Making the Decision

Colleges are out to get the best athletes. They play the recruiting game in sequence: the highest rated athletes get offers first; everybody else waits. Lesser name schools also wait as athletes hold on to see if big-time programs will offer them scholarships. The game has risks, both for the college and the athlete.

When you're deciding whether to accept an offer, lack of intelligence can be a problem. We're talking about intelligence as the CIA uses the word: information about the other side. You may not know what is in a recruiter's mind. They've offered you an athletic scholarship, but how many other offers have they made? How badly do they want you? Where do you stand with colleges that haven't yet made an offer but say they are interested?

Once again, the best way to find out is to ask. If you receive an early offer from a college that is not your first choice, ask whether you are *their* first choice. You may not always get a complete answer, but you can only gain by trying. You can also call a recruiter who has not yet made an offer and explain the situation. When you have an offer from one college, it puts pressure on the other recruiter to reach a decision about you.

Will the school you want more make an offer? Will the school that has made an offer still want you later? Once you've collected as much information as you can, make an estimate. Then take a deep breath, make the decision that seems right for you, and try not to second-guess yourself. Live with your decision and don't agonize over it. We all have to make decisions based on incomplete information. Some-times, no matter how carefully we think things through, a given situa-tion doesn't work out as well as we had hoped. But by not carefully thinking things through, we practically guarantee our own failure.

Deciding whether to sign early or late is one of the many decisions you have to make when selecting a college. It's good to weigh all the factors and make the tough decision. Taking control of your recruit-ment will not only help you select the right college: going through this process will also prepare you for success as an adult.

How Things Can Change after Signing an NLI

Gary Lawrence, a highly recruited football player, was offered a scholarship at a big-time football program in the Midwest at the beginning of the signing period, in early February. Gary had never visited the college, but the coach he wanted to play for was there, and the team was a powerhouse. Gary had heard rumors that the coach was considering an NFL job and that an NCAA investigation might turn up serious violations. He asked the coach about that, and the coach said he was staying at the college and the NCAA would find that his program was clean. So Gary signed the NLI as soon as he received it

Gary then learned from sports radio station KNUT that the coach had signed a contract with an NFL team. Later that day KNUT reported that the NCAA had banned the school from Bowl appearances for two years for serious recruiting violations.

Gary still had to go to the Midwest college or lose two years of eligibility, even though his reasons for attending that school were no longer valid. If Gary had waited until the end of the signing period, he could have played at other colleges. Gary, who hails from sunny San Diego, will ponder his mistake during the long, frigid Midwest winters.

Gary actually has alternatives. He could escape the jurisdiction of the NCAA by going to an NAIA school, where he would be eligible to play immediately. Attending a junior college would yield the same result. In either case, he could transfer to an NCAA program after two years.

PART FOUR

The College Years

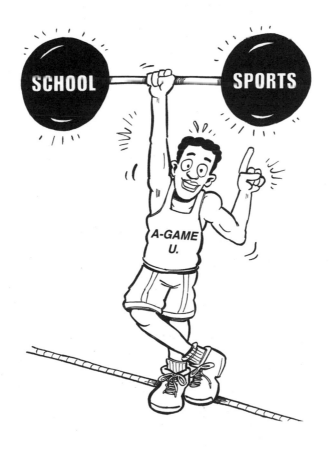

CHAPTER 14

Manage Your College Career

When you were a high school student, it may have been your mom who woke you up in the morning and urged you to hurry and get ready for school. While you took a shower, she prepared your favorite breakfast. As you inhaled her cooking, she reassured you that you were ready to do well on the math test. She would know: she had reminded you to study the night before. Then she put an overstuffed lunch bag in your hand as you rushed out the door.

The summer after high school flashes by—and suddenly you're in college. Your alarm goes off at 7 A.M., just in time to shower, dress, have breakfast, and make your 8 A.M. history class. But you were up late last night, and you've discovered the wonders of the snooze button (a feature moms don't have).

You hit snooze once, twice. You think, "I just won't take a shower, won't eat, won't look over my notes one last time." Then, a truly big thought comes into your head. "If I blow off this class, I could sleep for another two hours. My next class isn't until 10 A.M." Mom would call and make you get up if she knew what was going on.

College is a great opportunity. But where there is opportunity there is also danger. If you've prepared well in high school, you're ready to take advantage of everything college has to offer. But if you think college will be easy—or if you just don't think about it at all—you're setting yourself up for an upset.

College demands far more than high school. It's more competitive, both academically and athletically. You will do best if you assume college will be hard and bear down from day one. Get off to a good start and stay on top of your studies. If you let yourself get behind, it's hard to catch up. You'll feel overwhelmed and stressed out, and it will be hard to have a good time—even when you are playing your sport or relaxing with your friends.

Having said that, there's enough time to succeed in your sport and in your studies. Stay focused, you won't be overwhelmed by it all. If you manage your time well, you should even be able to have a social life.

College = Opportunity

College is a great place to develop your potential. Here's why.

- If you continue your sport in college, you'll be competing against the top athletes—in some cases, Olympic champions and future professionals.
- You learn to take charge. You decide what to major in, what career path to take.
- You are at a center of learning. You can take advantage of a concentration of knowledge, information, and ideas that exists nowhere else.
- You can get to know professors and students from many walks of life and see the world from their viewpoints.

Put it all together and your opportunities for a career and a meaningful, exciting, and enjoyable life as a college student are vastly increased.

Differences between College and High School

College will be new, but it's not a mysterious land totally unrelated to where you've been before. The skills you learned in high school are transferable to success in college. But it's important to understand some key differences between high school and college so you're prepared to deal with them.

No Roll Call

Many college courses do not require attendance. You can rationalize missing classes, but it's a formula for failure. Go to every class, pay attention, take notes. You will know what the teacher is focusing on, so you can study more effectively. Plus, it's easier to learn when you actively participate in class discussions.

More "Homework"

Much more. At college, they don't call it homework. It's assigned reading, exercises, writing papers, and preparing for exams. You may need to put in two, three, or four hours a day. Consistency is the key.

Longer Range Assignments

Some courses have reports due weeks or months down the road. Unless you devote time each day to the necessary reading or other preparation, by the time the deadline gets near, it's too late. Most courses have midterm exams on all the material covered to that point, and final exams that cover the entire course. It's impossible to prepare for these exams by cramming a semester's worth of material into a caffeine-induced, all-night study bender.

Harder Academic Work

High school courses often inch ahead, continually reviewing previous topics. College courses move at a quicker pace and cover more complex material. You can cruise along pretending everything is cool—until you take the final. Then, you take an F or you let your eyes wander to the test of the student to your right. Either way you have failed.

Parents Are Out of the Loop

In high school, your parents (or guardians) are expected to play a role in ensuring that you do your homework, fill out forms, pay required fees, return your library books. Each term your parents are invited to meet with your teachers to review your progress. If you're having an academic, attendance, or disciplinary problem, your parents are notified. In college, you are treated as an adult. You are responsible for your academic work and for completing all other requirements. If paperwork related to your financial aid has to be submitted by a certain date, it's up to you to make sure it's in on time. You can say, "I didn't know," but the college holds you responsible for knowing.

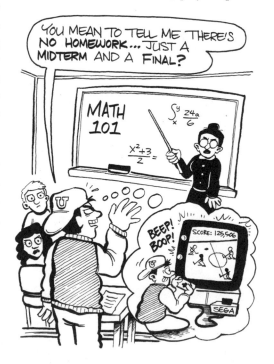

Increased Responsibility for Daily Life

For most athletes, college is the first experience living away from home. Many things you might have taken for granted in high school are now your responsibilities: housing, meals, laundry, housecleaning, paying bills, managing money, managing your time, deciding what courses to take. Even if you're still living at home while you go to college, you'll want the freedom and maturity that comes with taking care of your own business.

Harder Work in Your Sport

Perhaps you got by in high school as a "natural athlete." At college, you're up against the other "naturals." You're expected to put more time and effort into mastering your sport at a higher level. With practice, conditioning, film sessions, travel, and competition it can be the equivalent of a full-time job—even if the NCAA swears it's not.

Come Prepared

You wouldn't be the first person to arrive on campus and be quickly overwhelmed. All the new and tougher things about college hit you at once. It can be hard to know what to deal with first. Some college freshmen avoid dealing with any of it. They celebrate their freedom from home by hanging out and partying. Eventually the academic requirements catch up with them. At some point, just about everyone who goes to college thinks, "This is too hard—I'm leaving." If this happens to you, remember that most students who felt that way got their acts together and went on to accomplish great things.

As with sports, the single biggest difference between winning and losing is preparation. Those who have developed good habits in high school—eating and sleeping right, a disciplined approach to studying, an interest in reading and learning—tend to do well in college. They hit the ground running. Even if they stumble, they're trained to recover and keep going.

What If You're Not Prepared for College?

Many students—both athletes and nonathletes—arrive at college not ready to do college work. Some ignore the problem and hope it will go away. This only leads to flunking out. Other students identify their weaknesses and plug away at getting stronger.

Motivation can accomplish miracles. Even students who arrive ill prepared have overcome the problem and done well. It just takes a lot of hard work.

If you find you're not prepared for college-level work, deal with the problem. Take the remedial courses and special instruction you need to get you up to speed. The basic skills you need for success in college and beyond are the old three R's: reading, writing, and 'rithmetic—plus computer literacy.

Students who arrive unprepared but recognize the problem and work hard often do better than students who are complacent and think they will do well without applying themselves. Most coaches and employers will tell you that they prefer a hard-working person with some ability over a person who is a natural but doesn't maximize his or her potential.

Time Management, College Level

Your sport—including practice, physical therapy, weight training, watching films, team meetings, travel, and games—may take up to 40 hours a week. The NCAA restricts your coach to requiring no more than 20 hours a week from you, with additional time on a voluntary basis. "Volunteers" are the ones who tend to get playing time.

If you are taking a full schedule of courses, you will be in class 15 hours a week. There are 168 hours in a week. After classes, sports, and the time necessary for a good night's sleep and three meals a day, you're left with about 6 hours a day to brush your teeth, do the laundry, clean your room, socialize—and study.

You can do this if you manage your time efficiently. Review the techniques we covered in chapter 6 (see page 42).

The time you put into your sport is structured by the coach; studying has to be worked in around that. On any given day, you might finish a long and hard practice, take a quick shower, grab a bite, and then be faced with a decision. Do I shut my eyes for a short nap, or catch *Sports Center,* or get my butt to the library for three hours of study?

Plan to Plan

In college—with less structure than high school and no one holding your hand—planning is more critical than ever. To manage your time efficiently takes time, but a little bit goes a long way. You might decide that every Sunday at 8 P.M. you're going to spend 30 minutes planning your week and looking ahead to the following weeks and months. And that every morning you're going to spend 5 minutes reviewing the plan for that day and making necessary adjustments.

For most people, a plan isn't a plan until it's written down. The basics of time management are simple. Focus on what's important or urgent. If math is your biggest problem, make sure you schedule enough time to study math. If you're applying for summer jobs and the applications have to go out next week, schedule time to work on your resume right away.

If you don't schedule your time, you could work hard and still fail. It's like practicing hard but not smart: you could spend your time working on the wrong things. If you're getting good grades in Spanish, English, and history but failing math, chances are you're not budgeting your time correctly.

Make and Keep Commitments

We all tend to do things we're good at and that we enjoy and put off the tough stuff—those boring things we hate to do. Your plan says study, but you'd rather go out with your friends, watch TV, play a video game, sleep—anything but take care of the real business at hand. Once you've made your plan, be committed and carry it out. Refuse to be diverted. Your plan to study math at 8 P.M. is a promise to yourself. If you're tired, or if your friends are watching TV, your resolve may weaken. That's when you ask yourself, "Am I going to break this promise?"

Sometimes it's easier to keep a promise when other people are involved. For example, arrange to meet a friend at the library after dinner to study math. You're more likely to do it, even if you're tired.

Select a Major

Every college student has to decide what to specialize in. So you might major in history, computer science, biology, physical education, business, English, or any of dozens of other subjects. Particularly in your final two or three years in college, you'll probably take several courses in your major in each semester.

Some athletic programs steer you toward easy majors or even majors that are specially devised to keep athletes eligible. If you "major in eligibility," as this practice is called, you might end up with a college degree that represents little learning and is useless toward getting a job.

Select a major based on what you want to learn and what career you're interested in. Keep in mind that some majors may conflict with your sport more than others. For example, let's say you want to be a doctor. A pre-med major requires many laboratory courses in chemistry and biology. The lab hours may overlap your practice times. To pursue your sport and be a pre-med student would take careful planning. You might have to take some lab courses during the off-season, during the summer, or after you had used up your athletic eligibility.

When you begin in college you have a year or two to decide on a major. Use the same skills you developed when you selected a college: research and investigate your options; take elective courses in areas

---

To Transfer or Not to Transfer

Hopefully you've picked a school and an athletic program that are right for you and nothing is interfering with your enjoyment of your college experience. But what if you made a mistake in selecting a college or if things have changed—either with the college or with you—since you arrived? What if you are no longer enjoying your sport?

First, think the problem through; talk about it with coaches, advisors, parents, friends. Do everything you can to find a solution within the program. Transferring to another school is not an automatic ticket to happiness. You may find that the school you switch to is worse!

If you decide to pursue a transfer, there are rules that will govern your athletic options. If you are a Division I hockey player or basketball player (male or female) or a Division IA football player, NCAA rules require sitting out a year after you transfer. Some athletic conferences require sitting out two years if you transfer to another college within the conference. However, if you play football and you transfer from a Division IA to a Division IAA school, you are immediately eligible. In all sports, if you transfer from Division I to Division II or III, you are immediately eligible. Of course, if you transfer from an NCAA program to an NAIA or other non-NCAA school, you have escaped from all NCAA restrictions on your eligibility.

When you consider a transfer, there is another major issue—and perhaps the most important one: college academic departments often

---

you are considering as a major; ask questions. Your professors in departments you are interested in will be a good resource. Ask them about their courses, graduate school, and jobs in the field—and whatever else you need to know to choose wisely.

Take Charge

College is a key opportunity and, without the daily support of your family, it quickly becomes clear that your future is up to you. In this competitive world, no one has the main task of making sure you succeed except you. Coaches, athletic advisors, teachers, tutors, family, friends

don't accept all the credits you have earned elsewhere, and this can delay your graduation.

If your problem cannot be solved within your program, you've either got to live with it or make a move. In NCAA Division I or II, you must be released from your athletic scholarship to transfer and play in another NCAA program. Colleges are more frequently refusing to release athletes. Their position is that they have made a commitment to scholarship athletes and that it's not fair to the program for athletes to be free to leave on a whim. As we mentioned earlier, you could escape NCAA jurisdiction at an NAIA college.

This logic has holes in it. Athletic scholarships are renewable one year at a time, so a college's commitment has an element of, "What have you done for us lately?" And coaches can leave anytime, no matter how many years are left on their contracts.

Your college may say, in effect, that even if you don't like their food, you've got to stay and eat as long as they are putting it on the table. If you are determined to leave, however, they have to let you go. Slavery was abolished in the United States in 1863, even if some of the NCAA rules appear to bring it back. Sometimes the college uses its refusal to release you as a bargaining chip: "We'll let you go if you don't go to another school in the conference, or if you don't follow an assistant to the school where he is now head coach." Fortunately, most coaches understand that it's not in their best interests to stand in the way of an athlete who wants to leave.

will all help you if you seek their help. But you're in charge of your life. Ask yourself the following questions: What do you want? What must you do to get it? Who can help you? How will a small step today, combined with small steps tomorrow and the next day, lead to a breakthrough?

We've all heard motivational speeches that fire us up. But the next day, we might find ourselves sitting in front of the tube, aimlessly wasting time. Why does that happen? Because motivation that leads to consistent action comes primarily from within. We have to keep focused on our goals. And we have to develop the habit of tackling the tasks necessary to achieve those goals. The goal may be years away, but the satisfaction that comes from doing what needs to be done is a daily reward.

CHAPTER 15

Challenges College Athletes Face

College athletes face challenges that extend beyond athletics and winning. This chapter helps you overcome them.

Swelled Heads and Self-Doubt

A TV talk show host asked a star actor, whose husband is also a movie star, what their child thought about having two famous parents, "She's not impressed," the actor replied. "She thinks everybody's parents are on TV."

Maybe you were a star on your high school team. You were sought after by students who didn't even know if they liked you: they just wanted some of your glory to reflect on them. Teachers and administrators went out of their way to make things easy for you. Like the movie star's child, you may not have realized you were receiving special treatment.

At college you might continue to get star treatment; or you might find yourself suddenly spending a lot of time on the bench. Either way, some students and professors will think you do not have the brains to be at their school.

Don't rate yourself by what others think. You're who you are, whether others are foolish enough to worship you or sneer at you. Try to be objective about your abilities—athletic or academic—and work on improving them.

Broaden Your Horizons

As an athlete, you spend several hours every day with your teammates. You travel together and share a common interest in your sport. Naturally, your teammates will become close friends, and you'll value those friendships for a lifetime. But don't limit your circle of friends to athletes.

It may not be as easy to make friends with people who don't play organized sports, especially if you live in a dorm exclusively for athletes. But the extra effort is well worth it. When you spend time with people who have different experiences and attitudes, you receive one of the finest educational opportunities college has to offer: a chance to see how others view the world.

There's a famous line from Shakespeare's *Hamlet:* "There are more things in heaven and earth, Horatio, than are dreamt of in your philosophy." You don't need *CliffsNotes* to know Shakespeare got that one right. Today, more than ever, there is so much going on. Each of us is exposed to only a small part of it. In college you can meet people who grew up in New York City and Ulan Bator, and you'll have access to people who can open your mind to a vast range of knowledge—everything from astrophysics to zoology.

When it comes to making a circle of friends, don't limit yourself to people of the same race, religion, nationality, gender, or background as yourself. Hate and prejudice are passed down through generations of people who never bothered to see the world from the perspective of others.

On TV, complex historical, religious, and cultural questions are reduced to sound bytes. As a college student, you have the opportunity to sit down, talk with, and learn from people with different views. You can draw ideas from different cultures and areas of knowledge and incorporate them into your own life. Broadening your outlook will help you succeed in today's global society.

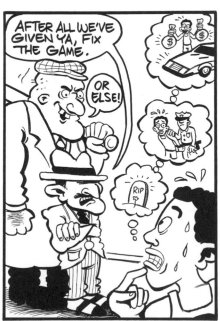

YOU BET YOUR LIFE

The World on Your Shoulders

If you're in a big-time college program that's getting media coverage, the emotional ups and downs of athletic competition can reach another level of intensity. Commentators and writers will describe games as though the fate of civilization depended on their outcomes. Boosters and fans will place the same importance on the games. You might find yourself, your coach, and your teammates glorified or denounced on TV, radio, or in print.

When the pressure is on, it's more important than ever to stay on an even keel and retain your sense of humor and your sense of proportion.

Gambling: A Tax on Imbeciles

Gambling is a huge problem in our society. It can be as addicting as alcohol or drugs.

In moderation, gambling can be controlled; after all, much of it is legal. You might wager a few dollars on a game of pool or the state lottery, or make a friendly bet on the big game. But if you're a competitive person (show us an athlete who isn't), once you start down that path, it can be hard to stop.

A couple of dollars wagered on a 2-on-2 basketball game can escalate into betting $50 on your favorite team. If you lose, we hope you realize when it's time to stop. Unfortunately, athletes tend to believe they'll win the next time out. In sports, this can be a great trait that can motivate athletes to learn and prepare better; in gambling, it's a formula for disaster.

An epidemic of gambling on sports is sweeping through college campuses, involving athletes and nonathletes alike. Many students go way beyond the occasional recreational bet. They squander their tuition money, their food money, their rent money, and they go deeply into debt. As they lose, they keep believing that they are going to come out ahead and beat the system. They haven't quite figured out where all the money to build those big hotel casinos in Las Vegas and Atlantic City comes from: gambling could be considered a tax on imbeciles!

Rules against Gambling

The NCAA prohibits college athletes from gambling on any sport. This means that a water polo player violates NCAA rules if he places a bet on a professional basketball game. If you are caught gambling on sports, the punishment is usually severe and can even mean permanent ineligibility. Gambling on sports is often treated more harshly than being caught with illegal drugs.

It makes no difference to the NCAA if the bet is made illegally through a bookie or legally through a Las Vegas sports book. And if you go to Vegas and lose your shirt on the slot machines or at the crap table, that's not a violation of NCAA rules (although it's certainly a rotten idea). But athletes are absolutely prohibited from gambling on sports.

The logic behind the NCAA's position is that college athletes and gambling on sports must be kept as far apart as possible to avoid any appearance that games might be fixed. Gambling on professional and college sports is a billion-dollar industry. In the real world, football and basketball are usually the only college sports on which there is widespread gambling, legal and illegal.

Point Shaving

Gamblers (often those with ties to organized crime) may try to entice you to fix a game by shaving points, a practice that is most prevalent in football or basketball. Or they may seek information from you about how prepared the team is or whether a teammate has recovered from an injury or illness. Your best strategy is not to provide anyone with team information that isn't already available to the general public.

Fixing games is not just a violation of NCAA rules: it's a federal crime, and it can put you in jail. Even if you are offered money by a gambler and you don't take it, but you don't report it, you are violating the law and the NCAA rules. If you're approached by a gambler, go to your coach immediately with the facts—even if other players are involved. Loyalty is a great quality, but people involved in criminal activities do not deserve your loyalty. The best tip we can give you is don't gamble your future by gambling.

Agents of Corruption

If you show potential to join the pro ranks as a football, basketball, baseball, hockey, tennis, golf, or track-and-field athlete, sports agents may try to develop relationships with you while you are still in college (or even high school).

Taking money or anything else directly or indirectly from an agent is a violation of NCAA, NAIA, and NJCAA rules. If you are caught, you will be suspended or disqualified. If you are caught signing a contract with an agent, you will be disqualified from competing in college. If you are caught taking money from an agent, the NCAA will deliver swift, severe, and terrifying punishment—such as the 29-game suspension of UCLA basketball player JaRon Rush during the 1999–2000 season. (Compare that to the two-game suspension of a football star who committed a felony.)

Agents are in competition to represent the few athletes who will become pros, and their prize is big: a percentage of a multimillion dollar salary and high-priced endorsement contracts. It's hard to know which players will make it to the pros, so agents try to develop ties with as many pro prospects as possible. Less scrupulous agents try to buy your friendship with parties, cars, cash, hotel rooms—whatever it takes.

College coaches want to keep agents away from college players, for agents have conflicting interests. Some agents—especially desperate ones with few clients—want athletes to jump to the pros as soon as possible so that agent can start taking his cut. Coaches want the best athletes to stay in school to keep the games exciting and the rankings high.

If you accept money or gifts from an agent and you don't get caught, there is still a big downside: you'll be in debt to an agent you've taken favors from. If you make it to the pros, you'll feel obliged to select that agent. But wouldn't you prefer an agent who spends time negotiating contracts for his or her athletes over one who gave you money and stroked your ego?

The Bottom Line for Dealing with Sports Agents

There is nothing wrong with talking to an agent, and there are many reputable agents who do not stoop to sleazy tactics. But as long as representing pro athletes is a lucrative business, there will be agents out to ensnare athletes in all kinds of overt and subtle ways. Don't think you can tell reputable agents from sleazy agents just by talking to them. When the time comes to select an agent, you will have to go through a careful process, just as you did when selecting a college. Meanwhile, as difficult as it may be—especially if you don't have two nickels to rub together—don't take anything from an agent. It may eat you up inside that others are getting rich off your talents. But why risk your college career for a quick buck?

When NBA player Marcus Camby was at UMass, he accepted money, clothes, cars, and stereos from two unscrupulous agents. He wasn't the only one: his family and friends did, too. When Camby didn't sign with either agent, they threatened to expose him and break his bones. Camby escaped physical damage, but he ended up reimbursing the agents. The NCAA stripped UMass from the 1996 Final Four record book and required the school to return $151,000. Camby repaid that sum as well.

Some agents use associates, known as "bird dogs," to get close to athletes. Bird dogs don't always say they represent agents. They may just start hanging around and befriending you. If you accept a gift, and it comes out that the gift-giver is associated with an agent, you pay the penalty; the agent or bird dog doesn't. The bottom line: there is no Santa Claus sliding down the locker room chimney. Agents give gifts to get something in return.

Boosters: The Ups and Downs

Supporters of the team may also offer you gifts, but it's a violation of NCAA rules to accept gifts from boosters. If you haven't much money and you suddenly find yourself among students who drive fancy cars and dress like they're from *90210,* it's hard to say "no" to gifts. And it may seem unfair, especially if you're on a team that brings millions of dollars into the school. Still, you're better off not accepting gifts from boosters. You put yourself in a position where you could be suspended or disqualified—and that's a big risk to take for a suit, an airplane ticket, or even a car.

There is something far more valuable than gifts that you can legally and ethically accept from boosters. Boosters tend to be prominent business and professional people. They can give you advice in their areas of expertise and leads to summer jobs and employment after graduation. A booster might even be able to give you a summer job in his or her own business.

Boosters may also be willing to provide you with personal references and letters of recommendation for graduate schools and jobs, as well as introductions to people who can help you.

Sometimes a booster will offer you a cushy job that's basically just a pretext to give you money. You're better off with a real job where you can learn something that will help you after you graduate.

Conflicts with Coaches

If you and your coach understand each other from the beginning, you can develop a great relationship and never have a significant problem. But things don't always work out that way. It's best to be prepared for conflicts with coaches, so if one does arise, you can handle it intelligently.

The Coach Tells You to Be a Team Player

When your coach tells you to be a team player, that's generally good advice. A group of athletes going after individual glory is a formula for failure. But what if your coach wants you to take easy courses that conflict with your educational goals? Or if your coach wants you to play in an important game despite a recent injury? (When it comes to injuries, don't hesitate to get a medical opinion from a specialist unrelated to the team.) The coach may talk about loyalty and sacrifice, but loyalty is a two-way street. Has the coach sacrificed any part of his or her agenda out of loyalty to you?

These situations can be complicated, and there are no pat answers. Sometimes it's right to make sacrifices for the team; sometimes your first loyalty must be to yourself. Use your judgment and seek advice from people you trust.

Don't Cheat Yourself Out of an Education

If you're having problems staying eligible and the team needs you, someone may offer to write your history paper or take your French exam for you. Everyone knows this happens; athletes and nonathletes get caught cheating every day.

Can a school have a championship athletic program without compromising its academic mission? The answer is "yes," but only if everyone involved—from the college president to the athletic director, professors, coaching staff, tutors, and boosters—are committed to playing by the rules. Everyone who's involved with the athletic department must strike a healthy balance between the desire to have a winning sports program and the necessity to provide the best possible academic environment.

What should you do if you're behind in your schoolwork and someone offers to cheat for you? It's tempting to accept such "help," for it may solve your immediate problems. And for every athlete who gets caught, there are dozens or even hundreds who don't. So why not take a chance if the odds are so good?

Because all students who cheat (including many nonathletes) get caught. First, they don't learn the material they will need for more advanced courses. Second, cheaters learn to look for the easy way out of difficult situations. The easy way out often leads to failed marriages, addiction, broken careers, even jail.

What looks easy can end up being very hard indeed. And cheating leads to more cheating. It's like lying: when you tell a lie, you have to tell another lie to cover up the first one.

Getting Help When You Need It

As soon as you realize you're having a problem with your schoolwork that you can't solve by yourself, search for help. Take advantage of the programs that are available and don't wait until you're failing.

Most colleges offer tutoring. If you're having trouble in a course, students who have mastered that subject can help you. There are often extra resources available—especially for athletes—including tutors, academic advisors, and counselors.

But be aware that there's a point at which tutoring crosses the line between helping you learn and doing the work for you. It's tempting to go along, even if neither you nor the tutor set out to cheat. Make it clear to the tutor that you want to learn. If necessary, go to the person in charge of the tutoring program and make sure you're assigned a tutor who will help you understand the material—not someone who will simply do the work for you.

Academic Requirements for Staying Eligible

For athletes to remain eligible, athletic governing bodies require athletes to be full-time students and to make progress toward a degree.

The NCAA, NAIA, and NJCAA define a full-time student as one who takes a minimum of 12 credits per semester. The NCAA also requires Division I athletes to comply with the 25-50-75 rule. This rule states that by the end of your second year, you have to have 25 percent of the requirements for graduation completed; by the end of your third year, 50 percent; and by the end of your fourth year, 75 percent.

The 25-50-75 rule recognizes that with the additional demands of your sport, it may take you five rather than four years to go through college. You are required to complete only one quarter of your academic work in the first two years, so the rule allows you time to adjust to college and take remedial courses if you need them. The rule still requires you to look ahead, beginning with your freshman year, and to make a five-year plan that keeps you eligible and leads to graduation.

Coaches and athletic departments want to keep you eligible, but their outlooks on how to accomplish that might be different from yours. Some programs are seriously interested in helping you learn; others just want you to stay eligible on paper for as long as possible.

They may steer you toward easy courses, some of which are especially created to keep athletes eligible. Going along with such schemes is just another way of cheating yourself out of a college education.

Remember that the courses you take and the major you choose at college are ultimately up to you. That major will prepare you for your future after college, so don't base such an important choice on what's easy in the short run.

CHAPTER 16

Prepare for Life after College

Life after college is the payoff for all the work you've been doing—from day one in high school, and even before that. Every word in this book has been written to help make your time in the "real world" rewarding. Not that it's ever going to be a piece of cake. But by now, we know you don't expect that. College was tougher than high school; the exams you will have to pass in your profession and as a spouse and parent will be still more challenging.

The key to success in college was early preparation in high school. Beginning in the ninth grade, you looked ahead to see what you had to do to be admitted to the college of your choice. You also found out what you needed to do to be eligible to compete in your sport once you got there.

Early preparation in college is also the key to success after graduation. If you're thinking about getting an advanced degree, what courses do you have to take to be eligible for graduate schools in your field? What entrance exams should you prepare for? If you intend to get a job immediately after college, what majors are employers in your field looking for? Are there summer jobs or internships that will help you be a highly qualified candidate?

The time to start thinking about these issues is in your freshman year, while there is still plenty of time to act on your decisions. "Are you crazy?" asked one stressed-out freshman. "It's hard enough just to go to practice everyday and keep up with my courses. I don't have time to dry off after I shower, let alone think about stuff four years down the road."

That's one way to look at it. But another point of view is that keeping an eye on the future will keep you motivated and help you decide which immediate demands are most important, which are secondary, and which are a waste of time.

I Don't Know What to Do with the Rest of My Life

Some students arrive at college with a precise career goal; they know they want to become a brain surgeon, an entrepreneur, an attorney. But you may not be one of these tightly focused whiz kids.

Don't worry: you are in the majority. Even students who traveled for a year after graduation, or those who hung out at their parents' homes until they were kicked out, have gone on to accomplish great things. We suggest that you view your uncertainty as an opportunity rather than a problem. College is the perfect place to explore career possibilities.

Talk to alumni and other students—especially juniors and seniors—about what their plans are and why. Take elective courses to find out if a field interests you and if you have an aptitude for it. Even if you have been certain since age six that you were going to be an electrical engineer, college is a great time to step back, ask yourself why, and investigate alternatives.

Statistics tell us you are likely to change careers at least once during your lifetime. Don't be afraid to explore new career ideas, during and after college. Even if you don't pursue those paths, the experience will be useful in whatever you do.

Careers in Sports

Many college athletes stay connected through their career choices. Most do not do it by becoming professional athletes. There are many other possibilities, including sports journalism, sports medicine, coaching and training, representing athletes as an agent or lawyer, athletic administration, radio and television production, and sports marketing. If you're interested in pursuing one of these fields, find out early in your college career what the prerequisites are. People you meet through your sport can be valuable resources. If possible gain experience as a summer intern. That will increase your employability and give a practical test of whether you really like the field.

Career Center

Your college will likely have a career center, or a place with the resources to help students prepare for life after college. This is a good place to explore career options, so become familiar with your career center as soon as you can.

There may be a library at your career center with information on exciting and rewarding careers that you never even heard of. Technology is changing quickly and new fields are constantly emerging. The 1970s and 1980s saw the advent of environmental law, sports medicine, sports psychology, and personal trainers—to mention just a few. In the 1990s, the Internet and World Wide Web and related careers become a major factor in commerce and in life. Executive coaching has also become a growing phenomenon. Business people and professionals have discovered what athletes have always known: a good coach can be vital to success.

Investigate all the resources available to you in the career center. In addition to information about careers, the center may include the following services.

- **Career assessment.** This involves testing to help determine what fields fit your values, skills, experience, interests, personality, and goals. You'll explore what your priorities are—whether they are making a certain amount of money or an opportunity to travel. You probably won't want a career in software engineering if constant tracking of thousands of details is not your thing. Career assessment will help you match your skills and interests with the right careers. Knowing what you want from a career and what you have to offer prospective employers will also be a strategic advantage in your job search.
- **Résumé preparation.** Your résumé is a key self-marketing tool designed to help you get a job interview. A résumé should present your skills, knowledge, and accomplishments relevant to your chosen career field—and it can even target a specific potential employer. If you have the opportunity to read sample résumés and cover letters and to get help from experts who have written hundreds of them, take advantage of it.
- **Mock job interviews.** An interview can be one of the big games of your life, yet many people go in with no practice. Your career center may offer to videotape your mock interview and review it with you. In an interview, you'll want to be prepared to answer questions about your qualifications and goals in a thorough, honest manner. You should also know how to deal with tough questions and be able to present yourself in the most favorable possible light.

Even more important than the technical resources of the career center are the people who work there. Get to know them. They can give you inside information about trends in the job market. They talk to recruiters (people offering jobs with paychecks) every day. Just imagine how nice it would be if, during one of those conversations, your career goals were on their minds and your name was on the tip of their tongues.

Online Job Services for Students

There are two Web sites that can help you in your job search.

- **StudentCenter.com** helps demystify the job-search process by emphasizing the importance of research and preparation. This Web site can help you identify your personal strengths, define your career goals, and fine-tune your résumé writing and interviewing skills.
- **JobTrak.com** is an electronic meat market (in the best possible sense, of course). It brings employers together with job seekers. In the old days, you would place your résumé on file in the career center. Recruiters would dig through piles of paper résumés to find candidates. Now everything's done online. Many schools use the JobTrak.com service exclusively. You post your résumé electronically so that recruiters can find it in the database.

Scoring Your First Job

If you were heavily recruited by college coaches, looking for your first job may be an eye-opener. Even if you have solid credentials, good grades, and strong extracurricular activities, you may be competing against many other well-qualified candidates.

In sports, your skills are relatively easy to showcase, but when you're seeking a job, you're judged more on things like your speaking ability and writing skills. Remember that a lot of the same qualities that made you successful in sports can lead to success in the business world. Communicate those abilities. Let potential employees know you're a leader and a team player; let them know you can take direction but you can also take initiative to start and finish projects. Package yourself to prospective employers so they can see that you are prepared for your career.

Here are some additional tips for landing your first job.

- **Pay attention to the details.** In your search for your first job, you may be asked to fill out formal application forms—especially if you are seeking a general, non-career-related position. Fill these forms out neatly and thoroughly, typing them whenever possible. Immediately after an interview, always send a thank you note to the interviewer. Spell the interviewer's name, his or her title, and the company name and address correctly. The best way to do this is to ask the interviewer for his or her business card. Paying attention to these details will often separate you from the pack. You might think no one would ever be foolish enough to misspell the name of an interviewer or company, but it happens frequently.

- **Get real world experience.** Anything you can do to acquire real-world experience makes you more valuable to an employer —and hence more marketable. If your schedule permits, seek an internship during the summer or academic year. Exposure to your chosen field may help you discover you'd really rather do something else—or that you like it even more than you expected. Boosters may be able to help you get experience in your field, through their own businesses or those of their friends and associates. Parents of teammates and other friends might be able to provide similar help. Don't hesitate to ask.

- **Be computer literate.** If you arrive at college without good typing and other computer-related skills, acquiring them while you are at college is a must. Computer literacy—including the ability to use the Internet—is fundamental in virtually every area of work today.

Keeping a Job, Then Moving Up

Like making the team, getting hired is just another beginning. To thrive in a competitive job market, you need to learn how to become increasingly more valuable to your employer, your associates, and your clients. Just as your coach determined your playing time based on your performance, so will your boss make decisions that impact your job responsibilities, opportunities, and salary.

Be proactive about your career. Many workers are content to sit back and believe that any new job skills they need will be taught to them by the company at the appropriate time. In the past, that may have been true. But lifetime employment with one company has become a rarity. In the incredibly competitive global economy, employers are looking to trim expenses whenever possible. When the time comes for the ax to fall, it will be too late for you to prove you're vital to the company's performance.

According to a study by the National Research Council, it now takes only three to five years for 50 percent of the average worker's skills to become obsolete. You need to improve your skills continually to make yourself valuable to a present or future employer. But this concept should come as no shock to an athlete: it's what coaches have been telling you since Day One. Don't rely on your good looks and sweet personality to stay employed. Be an expert in your job and know other people's as well, like a utility player on a baseball team who can fill in at many positions. In a business world that measures results, competence is a treasured commodity.

The idea of working full-time for one employer, particularly after you've gained some experience in your field, is no longer the only option. Today, many tasks are accomplished by strategic alliances of professionals who team up for a project and then break up after the job is done, perhaps rejoining for another project in the future. Even recent college graduates work as freelancers and start their own businesses.

The Value of Networking

As a college athlete, you're bound to be invited to functions at school and in the community: luncheons, banquets, award presentations, founding ceremonies, anniversaries of organizations, and so on. Athletes tend to look on these occasions as a burden. But if you focus on your future, you will see these affairs as opportunities. You are in a relaxed environment with successful business and professional people with whom you share a common interest. Rather than just sit with other athletes, approach these people and talk to them. Take an interest in what they do. (Even astonish your friends by talking to their parents.) These people will be delighted to get to know you, and they can be of great help to you after college. The old boy network is a terrible thing—until you (male or female) benefit from it. The reality is that job opportunities are based on merit *and* who you know. Preparing yourself to be strong in your field and developing a strong list of contacts is a powerful combination for success.

Networking after College

Virtually every field has at least one professional or trade association. It's never too soon to research these organizations and join the appropriate ones. You can learn a great deal and become more effective in your work; you can also make invaluable contacts.

In today's quickly changing workplace, you are likely to receive many short-term assignments. Through these assignments, you will meet a wide range of people at many levels—both those within and those outside your organization. Take advantage of the opportunity to get to know these people and weave them into your web of contacts. They may be in a position to help your career at some point in your future.

The A-Game Way on page viii counsels you not to settle for the minimum, on or off the field. This certainly applies to your profession. You may have an opportunity to pitch in and help your associates finish a project on time, even if it isn't your responsibility to do so. It might require sacrifices, such as skipping lunch, staying late, or even taking work home. But going the extra yard can demonstrate your ability and drive, and it can create a situation where people will want to help you.

Networking Is a Two-Way Street

The single best way to gain from networking is by helping the people in your network. The more you help them, the more they will view you as someone they want to help—and not someone who is pushy and always asking for favors. When you help one person, others find out about it and develop an appreciation for what you did. Pay attention to people's needs and wants and see where you can be of help. Early in your career, you may feel limited in what you can do. But it's amazing what happens when you put your mind to helping others. Suddenly you remember, for example, that your cousin Henry's company has a need for exactly the services that Jill, a person in your network, provides.

Have a Mentor

A mentor is a friend who is more experienced than you and willing to give you the benefit of that experience. Mentors can be parents, coaches, teachers, boosters, or other athletes. Whether you are still in college, starting a career, or working on an advanced degree, you need a mentor or two. Young people often avoid the company of older people and stick with their peers. Sometimes these young people talk as if they know everything and older people know nothing. What a way to rob yourself of the valuable experience older friends can provide!

Seek out mentors. They can help keep you focused and motivated when you're going through the rough spots. Many busy and successful people are willing to share what they know. It's not charity or a one-way street: successful people recognize the value of all the support and guidance they received along the way; they develop a need to give back to the community. And successful people benefit in many ways by surrounding themselves with up-and-coming young people, including staying in touch with new, emerging developments. Hopefully you'll look back on the people who helped you and you'll want to become a mentor yourself.

Getting into Graduate School

Whether you are planning to enter medical school, law school, or a graduate program in science or liberal arts, the graduate or professional school you're considering is likely to have admissions requirements beyond a college degree. There will be particular majors you must have, and even particular courses. Getting into the graduate program of your choice can be extremely competitive—like trying to break into pro sports. Special projects and extracurricular activities may enhance your credentials. Determine the requirements for graduate or professional programs as early in your undergraduate career as possible.

A mentor can be critical to your success. A professor in your department may provide tremendous help and encouragement in keeping you on track. Even as an undergraduate, consider joining the academic association in your field and going to its regional conferences and annual national meeting. These groups usually have reduced annual dues for student members.

By participating in the activities of your academic association, you may find yourself working and socializing with professors who will be evaluating your graduate school applications; this kind of contact can only increase your chances of admission. You may also be able to get published as an undergraduate, even if you simply participate in writing an article that appears on the Web site of an association. Publishing will also help your cause.

Good Luck!

If you concentrated on getting an education and not just a degree, and you took full advantage of your athletic experience, you will likely find yourself in the enviable position of having many options after college. You may be starting a challenging job or a graduate school program. Or you may even have the opportunity to continue your sport beyond college. Even if you're one of those select few, the skills you developed in college will prepare you for success in the business of professional sports.

Every athlete knows how important luck can be. A bounce can decide a game; an opponent's flu can decide a meet. But we did not include luck among the ingredients for success in chapter 2. That's because we know that if you steered clear of those shortcuts that turn into blind alleys, you've prepared yourself to make the most of the breaks that will come your way. We wish you good luck, knowing that you now have the tools you need for success.

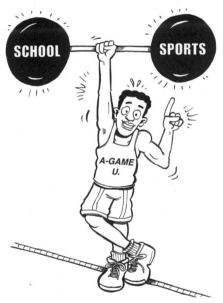

Postgame

by Mike Krzyzewski

Top college basketball programs are the focus of intense media analysis and commentary during the preseason. This hype puts unfair pressures on young people. College teams change too much for anyone to predict in September what the outcome will be in March. I tell my players that my only expectation is that they get better with each game.

Success means working hard, improving individual skills and teamwork, being part of something that's fun. It means developing trust and friendship and having an experience that will remain with our athletes for the rest of their lives. Success also means embracing education and graduating prepared for a career. We're proud of our Conference and NCAA Championships, and of our players who have gone on to the NBA. All of our hard work and teamwork led to those results. But there are over 300 Division I basketball teams, and each season only one wins the National Championship. Does that mean there are 300 failures? No. Teams that work hard and grow together as teammates and people are successful.

Reach Your Potential

It takes maturity to focus on working together for constant improvement, rather than dwelling on the most recent victory or defeat. The greatest thing an athlete, or any student, can accomplish in college is to become more mature and to develop the long-term outlook necessary for success. Maturity enabled our 1991 team to defeat UNLV on the way to the National Championship, after having lost to them by 30 points the year before. Maturity turns a good team into a great team.

What is maturity? The dictionary definition, "reaching full growth and development," works for fresh fruit, but I believe successful people never stop growing. I learn something about coaching from every practice and every game. At Duke, we try to recruit young men who are already mature enough to understand that they don't know all the answers. (That's important, as I don't even know all the questions.) These men are coachable because they want to improve. They listen, and they think about what they hear. They learn from mistakes.

Another part of maturity is taking responsibility for yourself and for your team and helping lead that team both on the court and off. As a coach, I am a teacher dedicated to helping my players be the best they can be—both in athletics and life in general. I am not, and I don't want to be, a policeman. We all make mistakes; I don't expect anyone to be perfect. But maturity is about understanding how your actions can affect your own life and your teammates' lives. Mature players tend to base their decisions on long-term goals rather than momentary gratification.

Numbers Don't Tell Us Who We Are

Selecting a college challenges a high school senior to become more mature. It's too easy to pick a college for an emotional reason: your friend went there, someone there says you're great, the team gets lots of TV exposure. It's easy to choose a school because of pressure from a parent, friend, or coach. This book shows you how to select the college that will best prepare you for the rest of your life.

The advice in these pages works, if you and your family put in the time to gather the information, weigh all the factors, and make a careful decision. When you're talking to the coach or making a campus visit, don't expect—and don't settle for—a magic carpet ride. Get a realistic portrait of the program, of life as a student there, and, most important, of the educational opportunities. When recruiting is based in reality and not hype, you and your future coach set the tone for an honest, open, trusting relationship that will benefit both of you for four years and beyond.

What sort of person are you? Think a minute before you answer. The answer has nothing to do with scoring 30 points a game, rushing for 1,000 yards in a season, or hitting 50 home runs. Those are numbers, but they don't tell us who we are. To perform well as an athlete, you need to develop qualities such as poise, teamwork, determination, integrity, selflessness. These are the same qualities that lead to success in any area.

Sports can be a funny thing. Sometimes chance, injuries, or even the way the ball bounces seems to determine the difference between winning and losing. But in the long run, hard work and preparation pay off.

Life is the same way. What do you do when you want success now but things don't go your way? That's the great test. Do you give up? Or do you dig down even deeper—knowing your efforts will be rewarded?

Sports can be your gateway to an education, a set of values, perhaps even a profession. Whatever your choices in life, remember that success is measured not by numbers but by maturity and character.

Good luck with selecting a college, and with having fun and getting a fine education once you are there.

Mike "Coach K" Krzyzewski is head basketball coach at Duke University. His Blue Devils won NCAA Championships in 1991 and 1992. He is the author of *Leading with the Heart: Coach K's Successful Strategies for Basketball, Business, and Life*.

Survival Guide for Parents

In addition to this section, we urge you to read the whole book. All the information in it will help you help your student athlete. If your child is still in high school, you will find part 3, The College Preparation Game, particularly relevant. Your son or daughter will especially appreciate your help with chapter 8, on financial aid.

As a parent of a young child, you have more influence than anyone else over how that child develops—even though there are days when you may not feel that way! As your child grows older, you will still play an important supporting role.

You can give enormous leadership, help, comfort, and inspiration to your child. Or you can add to your child's problems. We've all seen parents who make mistakes. Let's face it: sometimes we are those parents making the obvious errors. Just as you would want to help your child learn from his or her mistakes, learn from yours.

Having Fun Is Number One

Kids naturally play to have fun, and sports are organized ways to play. Kids can learn teamwork, discipline, concentration, goal setting, and sportsmanship from athletics—but only if they are enjoying it. The minute sports become a drag, a chore, or a source of anxiety, the experience changes into something that will hinder rather than help a child's development.

You can have a decisive role in making sports fun for your kids. Be there for them, especially when they are disappointed after a defeat (or what they perceive as a defeat). Tell your kids how well they played, how far they've progressed, how proud you are of the work they have put in and their good sportsmanship.

If you are involved in teaching your child athletic skills, be sure that you are doing far more encouraging than correcting. Kids do not want to constantly hear a list of their failings (neither do adults, for that matter). Children are not the only ones who want instant gratification; progress takes time and effort.

Don't Be a "Little League Parent"

Don't be the proverbial Little League parent: the parent who screams at their kids for making mistakes and screams at umpires and managers. These parents think that a 10-and-under Little League game between the True Value Cubs and the A&W Braves is the seventh game of the World Series. Little League parents can be found in any sport. They stress performance over participation. They think winning is everything, and they live through their children's success or failure.

If another dad or mom is acting like a Little League parent, tactfully point out how harmful this behavior is to their child and to all the other kids on the team.

Select the Right Coach

One of the best contributions you can make as a parent is to save your son or daughter from playing under a "Little League coach"—a coach in any sport, at any level, who carries on like a Little League parent. All good coaches believe in hard work, but the effort should be appropriate to an athlete's age and skill.

Some coaches motivate their kids by cursing at them, insulting them, and generally disrespecting them. Young athletes can be attracted to harsh, tyrannical coaches who have winning records. But no number of wins is worth the psychological damage that these negative types inflict on kids.

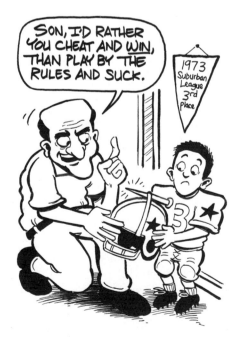

If your kid wants to play for a college coach of this type, understands what he or she is getting into, and is tough enough to handle it, that's one thing. But no kid should have to play for one of these monsters in high school or earlier;

and kids at that age don't have the experience to make an informed decision about that coach. The greatest coaches are people like John Wooden, patient teachers who love their athletes. They produce two kinds of victories: they win games and, more importantly, they mold athletes into mature and responsible adults.

Don't Be the Coach If You're Not

You know your kid better than anybody, so it's always tempting to advise the coach that your son or daughter should be playing more, or playing in a different position, or is better than someone else's kid. Imagine how you'd feel as a coach if every parent bombarded you with such suggestions. Once you've found a decent coach, be supportive, sit back, and enjoy the game. If you know enough about the sport to help your child learn a particular skill away from practice, that's fine. But don't set yourself up as the coach's competitor.

Listen to Your Kids

To help your kids, you need to know what's on their minds, what they are struggling over internally. Find out by listening more than talking, by asking more than telling.

Sometimes our kids tell us what they think we want to hear. It takes patience and understanding to get to the bottom of things. And we can't do that if we are busy imposing our identities on our children rather than helping them develop their own.

Parents should be courageous enough to ask their children why they are playing their sport. If the answer is not to have fun or if there is little enthusiasm, something is wrong. A good thing might have turned into a bad thing.

Imagine two friends who love basketball. They go out every day to shoot baskets and play in pick-up games; they play until it's so dark they can't see the rim. Both players get into an organized high school program, and they both look great on the court. But while one thrives on the pressure, the other one hates the pressure and finds that the sport he loved has become a miserable experience. The kid who now finds his sport a miserable experience may be afraid to say so—particularly if the parent projects the attitude that success equals being a star athlete and not competing means being a quitter. It can be a real struggle for parents to understand that their children may not feel the same way they do about sports.

A similar problem, which can also be an opportunity, arises when your son or daughter is faced with selecting a college. You may have strong feelings about where your kid should go. Maybe you strongly prefer one school: you went there, or you love the coach, or it's nearby, or it's got a great pre-med program. But to be helpful, you need to be open and listen to what your son or daughter wants to get out of college. You don't have to agree with your child, but if you don't seek out his or her views, your opinions will probably receive the same lack of attention.

Ideally, you and your child will be open with each other and you'll both come out of the discussion with more than you came in with. College selection and recruitment puts pressure on your family. Your ties with your son or daughter can get weaker or stronger: it's primarily up to you.

Your Help Will Be Appreciated

Kids need to be able to count on love and support from you, no matter what the circumstances. A parent best expresses that love and support by being open, by listening, and—if your child is open to advice at that time—by offering sound reasoning about what to do. If your kid doesn't immediately accept that reasoning, give him or her time to think about it. While it's good to be clear and firm about your convictions, nagging rarely helps.

Your son or daughter may dream of becoming a professional athlete. Maybe you share that dream. Working hard to achieve that goal can be productive and rewarding—unless it leads to ignoring academic and social progress. In this book we emphasize that out of the millions of youngsters engaged in sports, only a small percentage will become professional athletes. Every athlete, no matter how talented, is an injury away from the end of his or her athletic career. Concentrating solely on athletics is a foolish gamble that puts too much pressure on a kid and his or her family. Sooner or later, it takes the fun out of competing. As a parent, anything you can do to help your kid grasp this truth will be appreciated . . . eventually.

Important Questions to Ask Yourself

Keep in touch with your values and priorities to ensure that your actions serve your long-range goals. One way of doing that is to ask yourself a series of questions. We've developed questions that address athletics, academics, career, and the society around you. You may also have some of your own important questions to add to this list.

It is best to write your answers down, so you can refer back to them from time to time. But even simply thinking about these questions will help you set your priorities. When you need to make an important decision, look at your answers. See if you still feel the same way. Then make a decision that fits your answers.

Writing goals down can be a very effective way of turning them into a reality. Michael Jordan, Microsoft founder Bill Gates, and other successful people have written their goals on paper, reviewed them, and kept track of their progress. Written goals are a constant reminder of where you want to go. They help you avoid distractions and stay focused. (If you're still motivated mainly by money and not the journey, we should mention that Bill Gates is a multibillionaire; MJ isn't short of lunch money, either.)

These questions have no single, correct answer, and you may have multiple answers to many of them.

Athletics

- What am I trying to achieve? A career as a professional athlete? An Olympic medal? A successful and enjoyable time at college pursuing my sport? To be as good in my sport as I can?
- Why do I want this? Competition? Fun? Fitness? Fame? Money? Self- satisfaction?
- Do I like being an athlete and participating in my sport? What do I like about it? What do I dislike about it?

- What would I do if an injury prevented me from competing in my sport ever again?
- Am I learning values, habits, and skills from my sport that I can apply to other activities? What are they? Sportsmanship? Discipline? Working hard? Teamwork? Ability to think? How can I apply what I'm learning to academic work and to relationships with family and friends?
- Am I learning values, habits, and skills from academics and other areas outside athletics that I could apply to my sport? What are they?

Academics and Career

- Which subjects do I like? Why? Which do I hate? Why? How could I do well in those subjects anyway?
- What do I want to know about the world beyond sports? Why? Because it's better to know than not to know? To make a living? For the enjoyment of developing my mind?
- How do I want to earn a living? Have I considered alternatives? If I plan to be a professional athlete, how do I want to earn my living if that doesn't work out? If I don't know yet (which is perfectly natural in a young person), is it important to me to have a plan to find out? What's the next step in making a plan?

The Society around Me

- What are my values? Where do they come from? Philosophy? Religion? Family? Friends?
- Are family ties important to me? What kinds of relationships do I want to build with my parents (or the people who have been parents to me)? What kind of relationship do I eventually want to build with a spouse and maybe with children?
- Is it important to tell the truth? How do I feel about lying? What about cheating at school?
- Should I drink alcohol? Should I use drugs?
- What principles should govern my behavior with girlfriends or boyfriends? Am I ready to engage in sexual relationships?
- What do I believe now about social and political questions? How might my views change as I become older? Is it important to play a role in deciding social issues, to be involved in the issues affecting my community?

- What are my friends' good qualities? What qualities are not good? What kind of friends do I want?
- What are my good qualities? What qualities of mine are not good? What do I want to change? How can I do it? Who can help me?
- Do I consider myself a member of a community? If so, is that community my team, my school, my neighborhood, my country, my ethnic group, or the global community? Can I belong to more than one community?
- What do I want to get out of life?

The final group of questions about you and society is the most basic. If your answers to the sports and academics questions are not in line with your answers to the social questions, you've got some rethinking to do. Your answers, taken together, help you outline your goals. Select a college that will help you achieve those goals. Focus on actions that bring you closer to those goals.

Resources

Organizations

A-Game
P.O. Box 34867
Los Angeles CA 90034
www.A-Game.com

Free Application for Federal Student Aid (FAFSA)
800-433-3243
www.cd.gov/finaid.html
(Federal grants and loans)

National Collegiate Athletic Association (NCAA)
P.O. Box 6222
Indianapolis IN 46206-6222
317-917-6222
NCAA Hotline 800-638-3731
www.ncaa.org
Publications: *NCAA Guide for the College-Bound Student-Athlete; NCAA Guide for the Two-Year Student-Athlete; Making Sure You Are Eligible to Participate in College Sports; NCAA Transfer Guide; A Career in Professional Athletics: A Guide For Making the Transition*

NCAA Initial-Eligibility Clearinghouse
P.O. Box 4044
Iowa City IA 52243-4044
319-337-1492 (24-hour voice response service)
319-339-3003
www.act.org/ncaa/

National Association of Intercollegiate Athletics (NAIA)
6120 S. Yale Ave.
Suite 1450
Tulsa OK 74136
918-494-8828
www.naia.org
Publications: *A Guide for the College-Bound Student; Guide for Students Transferring from Two-Year Institutions*

National Junior College Athletic Association (NJCAA)
P.O. 7305
Colorado Springs CO 80933-7305
719-590-9788
www.njcaa.org
Publications: *Information for a Prospective NJCAA Student-Athlete*

National Small College Athletic Association (NSCAA)
113 East Bow St.
Franklin NH 03235
users.lr.net/~dmagee/

National Christian College Athletic Association (NCCAA)
P.O. Box 1312
Marion IN 46952
765-674-8401
www.bright.net/~nccaa

College Board (SAT)
P.O. Box 6200
Princeton NJ 08541-6200

609-771-7600
www.collegeboard.org

ACT
P.O. Box 414
Iowa City IA 52243-0414
319-337-1270
www.act.org

Collegiate Directories
P.O. Box 450640
Cleveland OH 44145
800-426-2232
www.collegiatedirectories.com
Publications: *The National Directory of College Athletics*

Web Sites

Preparing for college
A-Game, *A-Game.com*
College Edge, *collegeedge.com*
Collegiate Directories, *collegiatedirectories.com*
US News, *usnews.com/usnews/edu*
Yahoo!, *yahoo.com/education*

SAT and ACT
College Board, *collegeboard.org*
ACT Assessment, *act.org*
Princeton Review, *review.com/college*
Peterson's, *petersons.com*

Financial Aid
U.S. Dept. of Education, *www.ed.gov/finaid.html*
Finaid!, *finaid.com*
Fastweb, *fastweb.com*

Athletic Associations
NAIA, *naia.org*

NCAA, *ncaa.org*
NCCAA, *bright.net/~nccaa*
NJCAA, *njcaa.org*
NSCAA, *users.lr.net/~dmagee/*

Jobs and career
Job Trak, *jobtrak.com*
Student Center, *studentcenter.com*

General Interest
Initial-Eligibility Clearinghouse, *act.org/ncaa/*
Amateur Athletic Foundation, *aafla.org*
Amazon.com, *amazon.com*
CNN and Sports Illustrated, *cnnsi.com*
ESPN, *espn.com*
Life's Playbook, *lifesplaybook.com*
MyTeam, *myteam.com*
Leveledge, *leveledge.com*

Index

Visit A-GAME.COM

You've read the book. Now visit our Web site for additional information, insight and interactivity.

A safe harbor for athletes, parents, and coaches
A-Game.com empowers athletes by showing them how to avoid the traps and the sharks, and how to get the edge by relying on their own resources. It offers free, expert advice, based on the A-Game Way. It has information about the best products and services and about what not to buy: the dangerous, the shoddy, the overpriced.

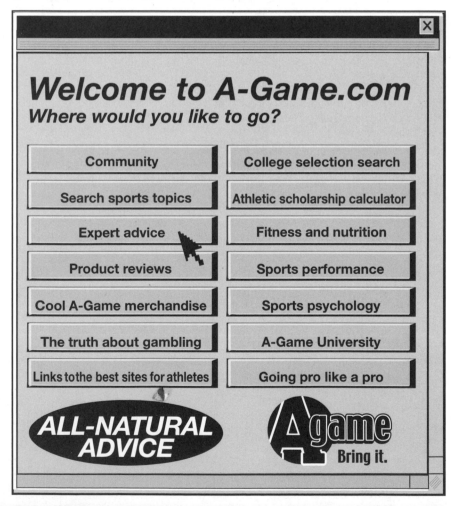

Welcome to A-Game.com
Where would you like to go?

Community	College selection search
Search sports topics	Athletic scholarship calculator
Expert advice	Fitness and nutrition
Product reviews	Sports performance
Cool A-Game merchandise	Sports psychology
The truth about gambling	A-Game University
Links to the best sites for athletes	Going pro like a pro

ALL-NATURAL ADVICE

A game Bring it.